# REIKI

# FOR BEGINNER

The ultimate guide to unlock the

healing power of Reiki

Respective authors own all copyrights not held by the publisher.

The information herein is offered for informational purposes solely and is universal as so. The presentation of the information is without contract or any type of guarantee assurance.

The trademarks that are used are without any consent, and the publication of the trademark is without permission or backing by the trademark owner. All trademarks and brands within this book are for clarifying purposes only and are the owned by the owners themselves, not affiliated with this document.

# Table of Contents

# INTRODUCTION

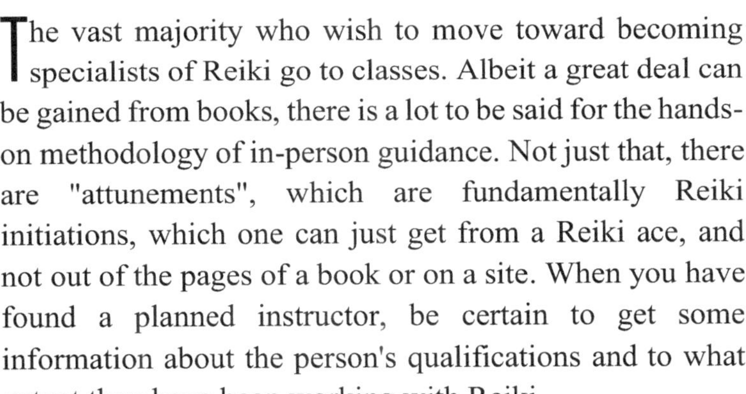

The vast majority who wish to move toward becoming specialists of Reiki go to classes. Albeit a great deal can be gained from books, there is a lot to be said for the hands-on methodology of in-person guidance. Not just that, there are "attunements", which are fundamentally Reiki initiations, which one can just get from a Reiki ace, and not out of the pages of a book or on a site. When you have found a planned instructor, be certain to get some information about the person's qualifications and to what extent they have been working with Reiki.

Among Reiki practitioners, there are fundamentally two camps: conventional and non-customary. The definitions change essentially, contingent upon who you inquire. Some consider that any individual who has strayed from the first lessons set out by Dr. Usui, originator of the Usui framework, is considered non-customary.

The book shows, tells and analyses the best way Reiki, as a healing process by touch, could help humanity. It reveals a cursory look at the perception and conviction of people towards the subject, thereby showing what it really is with practical examples.

This book is an offering for people and those searching the mystery behind Reiki. However, it shows how is best to administer it for optimal results of hand-healing which requires the transfer of vitality and energy to the body in need.

# CHAPTER 1
# INTRODUCTION TO REIKI

Reiki (pronounced RAY KEY) is a blend of two Japanese words, "rei" and "ki", meaning widespread life energy. Reiki is an old laying-on of hands recuperating procedure that uses the existent power vitality to mend, adjusting the unobtrusive energies inside our bodies. Reiki addresses physical, mental and profoundly irregular characteristics. This recuperating craftsmanship is a powerful conveyance framework. The Reiki professional fills in as a vessel that provisions recuperating energies where they are most required by the beneficiary. Reiki's ki-energies stream out of the expert's body through the palms of the hands while they are contacting the beneficiary's body.

## What's in store During a Reiki Healing Session

You will be asked to set down on a back-rub table, lounge chair or bed. You will be completely dressed, excepting your shoes. You may likewise be approached to expel or release your belt, so your breathing isn't limited in any capacity. It is ideal to pick baggy articles of clothing to wear upon the arrival of your arrangement. Wearing common textures is ideal (cotton, fleece, or cloth). You may likewise be approached to expel any adornments (rings, arm ornaments, pendants, and so forth) preceding the session, so think about leaving these things at home.

### Loosening up Atmosphere

Reiki experts will regularly make a loosening up air for their Reiki sessions, setting the state of mind with the utilization of darkened lights, thoughtful music, or foaming drinking fountains. A few professionals want to be in a spot that is totally quiet, without the diversion of music of any sort, to lead their Reiki sessions in.

### Recuperating Touch

During the Reiki recuperating session, the expert will put his hands gently on various pieces of your body. Some Reiki professionals will pursue a predetermined sequence of hand situations, enabling their hands to lay on each body area for 2 to 5 minutes before proceeding onward to the following. Empathic experts will openly move their hands in no specific order to the regions where they "feel" Reiki is generally required. Some Reiki specialists don't really touch their customers. Rather, they will drift their lifted palms a couple of crawls over the leaned back body. In any case, Reiki energies stream where they are assumed to. Reiki is a savvy vitality that consequently streams where the lopsided characteristics are in your body paying little respect to where the specialist's hands are put.

## Apparition Hands

Since Reiki energies stream to where they are most required, there is a Reiki marvel called phantom hands that you could be possibly understanding. Ghost hands feel as though the Reiki specialist's hands are contacting one piece of your body when they are placed elsewhere. For instance, you might have the option to see that the healer's hands are really set on your stomach, however you could swear that hands are touching your legs. Or, on the other hand, you may feel a few sets of hands on your body simultaneously, as though a few people are in the room with you.

## Booking a Reiki Healing Session

You may have gone to the business catalog or your phone registry looking for a Reiki expert in your general vicinity. In any case, not many professionals publicize their administrations utilizing the media. Reiki specialists work in centers, emergency clinics, spas and self-started ventures. A few specialists give house-calls, venturing out to your area to give medicines. Look at announcement board postings in common markets, powerful stores, yoga classes, junior colleges and so forth. Reiki specialists frequently depend on verbal exchange from their customers to get in contact to new ones.

And there is a wide range of Reiki frameworks, so make sure to pose any inquiries you may have about a professional's consultation before you book a session.

Reiki shares are now and always have been utilized as a limited time instrument to present Reiki in their regions. Offers are normally made intermittently week-ends for nothing or at a negligible cost.

## Turning into a Reiki Practitioner

Reiki is customarily studied in three levels. Level I and level II are regularly instructed in one day classes (8 hours) or over an end of the week time frame (16 hours). Level III is for the most part a progressively serious course of study and will take a more drawn out responsibility. Class time includes an inception called an attunement and learning the hand placements for self-treatments as well as treating others.

## Reiki Controversies and Myths

The mending network has progressed significantly in demystifying the shroud of mystery that once encompassed the instructing of Reiki in the western half of the globe. Accordingly, errors that were resulting from the educating being shrouded away, have been worn down layer by layer. Be that as it may, some of these Reiki Myths continue to develop naturally.

Reiki was first acquainted with Canada and the United States in the 1970s. Hawayo Takata, a Hawaii local of Japanese drop, brought her insight into Reiki to the territory through verbal lessons. Reiki lessons and stories were passed down from educator to understudy by listening to others' conversations for quite a long while. No big surprise the narratives got cluttered up! There is a proceeding with contention about publicizing the symbols used in Reiki. They have been discussed as being sacrosanct and ground-breaking and ought not be shared outside of the Reiki people group. However, the images are imprinted in a few productions and broadly conveyed over the Internet. What may have stayed quiet for a moment will never again. I, for one, don't accept that images have control of themselves, however that the power they speak to is really the expectation or center held by the Reiki specialist when they are being utilized.

Reiki originates from two Japanese words which mean "widespread life power." This all-inclusive life power is a vitality found inside all things—individuals, creatures, plants, rocks, trees... even the Earth itself. Somebody prepared in the utilization of Reiki channels uses that life power, enabling the beneficiary to recuperate their vitality.

**Eastern Methods, Western Medicine**

This mending methodology came to us from Japan, however Western medication is at long last starting to perceive its advantages. Real therapeutic centers, including the emergency clinic at Ohio State University, are currently finding the estimation of integrative mending—at the end of the day, conventional Eastern recuperating techniques are utilized to supplement present day prescription.

### Images and Spirit Guides

Some portion of Reiki treatment incorporates the utilization of holy images. In certain conventions, these are kept quiet from any individual who hasn't started into the framework. In different ways, a few images have been made public for books and the Internet. Notwithstanding the images, nonetheless, a Reiki expert may call upon spirit guides, rose masters, or holy messengers, contingent upon their profound way. Reiki isn't a religion and individuals from a wide range of beliefs practice it.

### Mending Energy

In Reiki, mending happens on an enthusiastic, otherworldly and physical level. The professional spotlights on the recipient's Chakra systems. Here and there, these uneven characters appear because of physical illnesses—a cerebral pain, a stomach infection, and so forth. In different occasions, it might be identified with a type of passionate or otherworldly issue that the individual hasn't settled at this point—relationship issues, issues at work, outrage at a parent or life partner. By moving Reiki vitality into the beneficiary, the expert can enable the person to recuperate through whichever issues are nearby.

## The Merits of Reiki

Reiki can be utilized to treat various infirmities, both physical and mental. As per its creator, Dr. Mikao Usui, only a couple of the numerous advantages of Reiki are:

· Treating passionate injuries from prior throughout everyday life

· Giving quieting vitality to somebody who might be overpowered by pressure

· Cleansing food or drink by gifting them with Reiki vitality

· Using it paired with ordinary wellbeing practices and medication

· Improving or amplifying spiritual mindfulness

· Mitigating torment brought by illness or damage

· Giving restorative alleviation to somebody who might mourn a misfortune

## What Reiki isn't:

A religion—Assuming you study Reiki, you won't be approached to revere a specific divinity, nor will you be approached to surrender your present religion. Reiki can work paired with your otherworldliness, yet doesn't supplant it.

A substitute for restorative consideration from a doctor—if somebody has an ailment that requires treatment, they have to see a specialist. A Reiki professional can help with anguish and recuperating enthusiasm, however, ought to never decide.

Back rub treatment—somebody searching for remedial back rub should see an authorized massage specialist.

However, The International Center for Reiki Healing says, "While Reiki is profound in nature, it's anything but a religion. It has no doctrine and there is nothing you should provide in order to learn and utilize Reiki. Truth be told, Reiki isn't reliant on conviction at all and will work whether you provide or not. Since Reiki originates from God, numerous individuals find that utilizing Reiki places them more in contact with the experience of their religion as opposed to having just a scholarly idea of it."

## What's in store in a Reiki Session

Assuming you've booked a Reiki session, this is what you can expect: a regular Reiki specialist will have you lay on a table, the goal being for you to be completely relaxed and to enjoy the experience. You don't need to take off your garments for Reiki to be compelling. Usually, there will be delicate music playing and the lights will be muted, so that you can unwind. Your Reiki specialist will utilize an exceptionally light, non-obtrusive touch to work with your vitality. You may nod off during your session, experience changes in temperature, or even feel an extreme flood of feelings; a few people burst into tears during Reiki. These are typical encounters, so don't be frightened assuming they occur.

Once your session is finished up, you will doubtlessly feel invigorated and have a recharged feeling of lucidity. Make certain to remain hydrated during your session.

Reiki is a Japanese system dependent on the (logically demonstrated) premise that there is a Universal Life Energy in every living thing. The Usui System of Reiki recuperation applies this vitality through touch to mend. A Reiki Practitioner puts their hands on the patient and transmits high recurrence vitality into them to address lopsided characteristics in the body. Reiki works in amicability with every other type of healing and is routinely utilized in medical clinics and centers.

**Why have a Reiki treatment?**

Hands on mending has been deductively demonstrated to be successful in quickening healing. A Reiki treatment underpins the entire individual including body, feelings, psyche and soul, making numerous helpful impacts. On a physical level Reiki enables agony reduction, accelerates the amelioration time of bones and wounds, loosens up muscles and diminishes the tissue damage. It is conceivable to decrease the negative symptoms of medicines, for example chemotherapy and radiation. Colds, flus, honeybee stings, coronary illnesses -

numerous physical conditions can be treated with Reiki. On a psychological level uneasiness is diminished, a feeling of prosperity expanded and another degree of unwinding felt. At this level of profound unwinding a rebalancing of energies happens and the normal recuperating capacity of the body is upgraded. On a spiritual level, subjects have expressed that they feel renewed and revived after a full-body session. How is a Reiki treatment given?

A common Reiki treatment will have the patient lying full dressed on a back rub table. It is likewise conceivable to give a Reiki treatment to a customer sitting or standing. The professional places his or her hands on or close to the customer's body in a progression of hand positions from the head to the feet that are held for somewhere in the range of 2 to 10 mins, contingent upon how much time is required at each hand arrangement. The treatment will commonly last somewhere in the range of 45 mins to an hour and may incorporate criticism acquired by the expert during the treatment. A customer may profit to their specialist for every other week reason for some time or may locate that one session gives all the important advantages. Reiki specialists are able to offer long distance sessions, so you could be anyplace on the planet and get mending from your professional.

## Reiki treatment: What it feels like for those who undergo it

Everybody will have a somewhat extraordinary encounter, anyway ordinary individuals might feel an amplified feeling of unwinding. By and by, you'll feel a stunning shining brilliance or vitality traveling through your body, in some cases in floods, and it will course through you and surround you. Others will have dreams, or feel like they are skimming over their body. Where the expert feels blockages in a customer's vitality (and will invest time clearing that blockage) the customer may feel an underlying weight, however, then a discharge and stream of vitality. It isn't surprising for clients to encounter a passionate discharge as an enthusiastic disturbance is brought to the surface and discharged.

Reiki is likewise an otherworldly practice that develops genuine feelings of serenity, upgrades our wellbeing and imperativeness and advances mental prosperity. Day after day self-Reiki medicines are looked for more and more: the foundation of thinking more about ourselves and developing validation and wellbeing on all levels. Reiki is the blessing that continues giving.

The word "Reiki" implies soul vitality or the vitality of the Universe, which is found in every single living thing, plants and creatures notwithstanding. As people, we are altogether brought into the world with Reiki; an attunement or reiju** is everything necessary to enable us to enact or stir this capacity and recall all that we can do.

The training started with Mikao Usui in Japan back in the mid-1920s. Usui's understanding of illumination and deep-rooted profound practice drove him to build up the recuperating strategy we currently know as Reiki. He created Reiki as an otherworldly practice to develop true serenity in this way advancing wellbeing and prosperity. Usui Sensei skilled us with the Reiki statutes as instruments for mental prosperity and profound development.

**A portion of the advantages of Reiki may include:**

· Abatement in agony and tension;
· Helping the body in clearing poisons (for example, chemotherapy or radiation);
· Adjusting body, brain and soul;
· Stress decrease; unwinding;
· Improvement of wellbeing and prosperity; rebuilding of imperativeness; self-care;
· Upgrading and quickening the ordinary healing procedures of the body;
· Upgrading the body's capacity to recoup from wounds, medical procedures, or injuries;
· Help from physical and mental impacts of pressure;
· Reiki is sheltered. It is non-pharmaceutical, non-obtrusive and moves one towards parity.

There are no known contra-signs (reasons not to give) and no known reactions despite this fact, the adjusting and mending procedure can deliver transient uneasiness.

Reiki can be utilized by individuals for all things considered; from pregnancy for the duration of the life expectancy. Creatures likewise love Reiki and many pet owners currently offer Reiki to their dearest pets.

Reiki doesn't meddle with any customary medicinal treatment or prescription you might get. In view of its unwinding impacts and in general benefits, a few people may find that they may require less medication. Any drug modification ought to be made under the supervision of their primary care physician.

**How Does Reiki Work?**

We don't have the foggiest idea about the accurate instrument of activity of how Reiki functions, however it appears to initiate the unwinding reaction. At the point the body is loose, the reactions of stress are diminished. Furthermore, similarly as Florence Nightingale, the author of the advanced nursing convention portrayed how the job of the medical attendant is to "… placed the patient in the best condition for nature to follow up on him," by realizing the unwinding reaction, Reiki expels physiological worry from the body and the body does what it was intended to do—mend itself and come back to adjust.

## How is a Reiki Session?

A Reiki session is generally led in a calm room, where the individual would sit in a seat or lay on a back-rub table or chair. Delicate loosening up music would play out of sight. A general session would incorporate setting hands on or simply above different areas on the body (these positions are situated close to the significant organs of the body). This could incorporate the head, front and the back of the body. A Reiki session could likewise be centered around only a couple of regions of concern, damage, agony or uneasiness. The session would be as long or as short as required. A short, engaged session can last from 10 to 40 minutes and a full body session can last from 45 to an hour and a half. All the individual needs to do is unwind and get the mending vitality. Talking is normally not empowered so the individual can get the full advantages of unwinding.

Reiki is easy to use and can be adjusted to and utilized in any setting; home, clinic, hospice, creature sanctuary or clinic, medicinal workplaces, testing bases, crisis settings and numerous others.

# CHAPTER 2
# HISTORY OF REIKI

The Reiki strategy for heling was established on the disclosure and comprehension of the body's vitality framework. Reiki Practitioners endeavor to improve wellbeing and personal satisfaction by offering Reiki vitality and reestablishing harmony. Reiki is utilized in self-care, for consideration of one's family and is offered in private practice, in emergency clinics and restorative environments as an aide and steady treatment to health and conventional medicinal consideration. The type of Reiki that numerous individuals practice today, Usui Reiki, has been used for more than one hundred years.

## The Founder of Reiki

The historical backdrop of Usui Reiki starts with its founder, Dr. Mikao Usui. Now and then called the Usui Sensei, Dr. Mikao Usui was born in a well-off Buddhist family in 1865. Dr. Usui's family had the option to give their child balanced instruction for that time. As a tyke, Dr. Usui grew up in a Buddhist religious community where he was shown hand to hand fighting, swordsmanship, and the Japanese type of Chi Kung, known as Kiko.

All through his training, Dr. Usui had an enthusiasm for medicine, brain research and religious philosophy. It was this intrigue that incited him to look for an approach to heal himself as well as other people utilizing the laying on of hands. It was his longing to discover a curing technique that was unattached to a particular religion and religious conviction, so his framework would be available to everybody.

Dr. Usui voyaged a lot during his lifetime. He concentrated mending frameworks of various types and held various callings including journalist, secretary, teacher, community worker and watchman. At long last, he turned into a Buddhist cleric/priest and lived in a religious community.

## Otherworldly Awakening and Development of Reiki

At some point during his long stretches of preparing in the religious community, Dr. Usui went to his very own preparation rediscovery course in a cavern on Mount Kurama. For 21 days, Dr. Usui fasted, contemplated and prayed. Moreover, on the morning of the twenty-first day, Dr. Usui encountered an occasion that would change his life for eternity. He saw old Sanskrit images that helped him build up the arrangement of healing he had been attempting to design. Usui Reiki was conceived.

After his otherworldly awakening on Mount Kurama, Dr. Usui built up a facility for curing and educating in Kyoto. As the act of Usui Reiki was spreading, Dr. Usui ended up being known for his healing practice.

**Other commendable Development about Reiki**

Hands on mending has been logically demonstrated to be viable in speeding up healing.

A Reiki treatment bolsters the entire individual including body, feelings, brain and soul making numerous helpful impacts.

On a physical level Reiki enables reduction of pain, quickens the mending time of bones and wounds, loosens up muscles and decreases the tissue formation on wounds. It is conceivable to ameliorate the negative symptoms of medication, for example, chemotherapy and radiation. Colds, flus, honeybee stings, coronary illness - numerous physical conditions - can be treated with Reiki.

On a psychological and passionate level uneasiness is diminished, feelings of prosperity expanded and another degree of unwinding can be felt. At this level of profound unwinding a rebalancing of energies happens and the common mending capacity of the body is improved.

On a spiritual level, patients have expressed that they feel reawakened and restored after a full-body session.

## How is a Reiki treatment given?

A run of the mill Reiki treatment will see the customer lying fully dressed on a back-rub table. It is additionally possible to give a Reiki treatment to a customer sitting or standing. The professional places his or her hands on, or close to the customer's body in a progression of hand positions from the head to the feet holding them for 2 to 10 mins, depending upon how much time is required at each hand arrangement. The treatment will commonly last somewhere in the range of 45 mins to an hour and may incorporate input acquired by the expert during the treatment. A customer may refer to their professional for a fortnightly appointment, for some time or may find one session enough for all the vital advantages. Reiki experts are able to give separation mending, meaning you could be anyplace on the planet and get healing from your expert.

## What does a Reiki treatment feel like?

Everybody will have a somewhat extraordinary encounter. Anyway, regularly, individuals experience a stronger feeling of unwinding. I, personally, feel a stunning sparkling brilliance or vitality traveling through my body, here and there in floods and it will move through me and surround me. Others will have dreams or feel like they are drifting over their body. Where the specialist feels blockages in a subject's vitality (and will invest time clearing that blockage), the patient may feel an underlying largeness followed by a discharge and stream of vitality. It isn't unusual for customers to encounter a passionate discharge, as enthusiastic disturbance is brought to the surface and discharged.

Reiki is likewise a profound practice that develops genuine feelings of serenity, improves our wellbeing and essentialness and encourages mental prosperity. Every day self-Reiki medication is an attraction of health: the foundation of thinking about ourselves and attracting consistency and wellbeing on all levels. Reiki is the gift that keeps on giving.

The word "Reiki" implies soul vitality or the vitality of the Universe, which is found in every single living thing, plants and creatures notwithstanding. As individuals, we are altogether brought into the world with Reiki; an attunement or reiju is everything necessary to enable us to actuate or stir this capacity and recall all that we are able to do.

The training started with Mikao Usui in Japan back in the mid-1920s. Usui's involvement of illumination and deep-rooted profound practice drove him to build up the healing technique we currently know as Reiki. He created Reiki as a profound practice to develop significant serenity in this way expanding wellbeing and prosperity. Usui Sensei skilled us with the Reiki statutes as devices for mental prosperity and profound development.

The Reiki strategy for healing was based on the disclosure and comprehension of the body's vitality framework. Reiki Practitioners endeavor to improve wellbeing and personal satisfaction by offering Reiki vitality and reestablishing harmony. Reiki is utilized in self-care, for consideration of one's family and is offered in private practice and in emergency clinics as an assistant and steady treatment to wellbeing and customary medicinal consideration. The type of Reiki that numerous individuals practice today, Usui Reiki, has been used for more than one hundred years.

As we stated, the historical backdrop of Usui Reiki starts with its originator, Dr. Mikao Usui.

In the mid-1990s there were discoveries of Usui's unique Reiki lessons. The commemoration of Usui was found by western instructors and many people from Reiki's missing connections were revealed. Disclosures incorporated the revelation of a living Reiki practice in Japan, with extra strategies as instructed by the Reiki Gakkai (Reiki Learning Society). Some of Usui's notes and manuals were likewise shared and this prompted more noteworthy discoveries which were later made and became largely accessible. Western Reiki instructors increased new data seeing the framework as it had been taught in Japan and this was sorted out with set up frameworks of Reiki in the West.

## Usui's Students

On September 1ˢᵗ 1923, the devasting Kanto earthquake struck Tokyo and the surrounding regions. A large portion of the center piece of Tokyo was leveled and completely pulverized by flame. More than 140,000 individuals were murdered. In one case, 40,000 individuals were burned when a flame tornado cleared over the open territory where they had looked for shelter. Tragically the quake struck in the late morning, exactly when peoples' charcoal flame broils were set to prepare lunch. 3,000,000 homes were shattered, leaving endless amounts of people broke. More than 50,000 individuals endured serious wounds. The open water and sewage frameworks were destroyed and it took a very long time for re-working to happen.

Considering this disaster, Usui and his students offered Reiki to numerous unfortunate casess. His facility turned out to be too little to even consider handling the crowds of patients, so in February 1924, he manufactured another center in Nakano, outside Tokyo. His notoriety spread rapidly all through Japan and he started accepting solicitations from everywhere throughout the nation to come and show his healing techniques. Usui was granted a Kun San from the Emperor, which is a high grant (much like a privileged doctorate), given to the individuals who had done respectable work. His acclaim before long spread all through the district. Numerous noticeable healers and doctors started mentioning lessons from him.

Usui rapidly turned out to be head over heels as solicitations for instructing Reiki kept on arriving. He travelled predominantely all through Japan which was not a simple endeavor back then, to instruct and give Reiki attunements. This began to negatively affect his wellbeing and he started encountering light strokes from pressure. On March 9th, 1926, while in Fukuyama, Usui unfortunately died of a lethal stroke. He was 62 years old.

It is said that Usui instructed Reiki to a little more than 2000 individuals and out of these successors a few sources state he prepared 22 to educator level(Shinpiden). Huge numbers of these students started their very own centers and established Reiki schools and social orders.

By the 1940s there were around 40 Reiki schools spread all over Japan. The vast majority of these schools taught the strategy for Reiki that Usui had created.

## Dr Chujiro Hayashi

The ancestry of most of Western Reiki experts springs from Chuijro Hayashi. Hayashi taught with Mikao Usui for around ten months preceding Usui's passing. He is known to have changed a portion of the strategies of Usui.

Chuijro Hayashi was born in 1879. At some point, in 1925 Chuijro Hayashi met Usui. Chuijro had ascended to be an authority in the Imperial Navy and had prepared in Western and Chinese Medicine. In June of 1925, Hayashi got his instructor's preparation in Usui's framework. A few sources state that Chuijro Hayashi was a Methodist Christian, a reality affirmed one of his Shoden/Okudent understudies, Mrs.Yamaguchi. Different sources state that he was a Soto Zen specialist who used the acts of Shinto. For all we know, he may have been both as this would be flawlessly as per Japanese ways to deal with religion. As a Christian, Hayashi would have taken in the rearranged type of Reiki.

Before his demise on tenth May 1940 Hayashi coached 13 students to the educator level, inccluding Hawayo Takata in 1938.

## Mrs. Takata - Usui Shiki Ryoh

Hawayo Kawamura (her original last name) was brought into the world on December 25th 1900 in

Hanamaula, Kauai, Hawaii. On the tenth of March 1917 she married her significant other, Saichi Takata. They had two little girls, one named Alice Takata-Furumoto, who later had a little girl named Phyllis Furumoto.

It is because of Mrs. Takata that Reiki is outstanding and wide spread all through the world. Mrs. Takata officially brought Reiki to America at the beginning of the 1970s and during a multiyear time frame, brought 22 Western students to the instructor level. Her style of Reiki was created from the learnings she recieved from Dr Hayashi.

It was following the death of her significant other in 1930 and her sister's in 1935 that Hawayo Takata chose to go to Japan to visit her folks. Because of the work she put into help her family and the sadness caused by her loses, Takata's wellbeing had started to suffer. She has booked an appointment in Japan to check her medical issues. Just before the appointmen she heard the voice of her dead spouse, saying that the practice she's chosen was a bit much and that there was another way. This determined her to talk with her primary care physician about elective medicine, so he suggested her Hayashi's Reiki Clinic. Hawayo Takata gotten day by day medications at stayed at this facility for a period of four months and during this time her symptoms totally subsided.

This drove Hawayo Takata to take Reiki One preparing (Shoden) with Hayashi on December 10th, 1935. She examined the principal level with him for barely one year. In 1937, Mrs. Takata got the subsequent level, Okuden. Soon after this, she came back to Hawaii. Half a month later, Hayashi visited Mrs. Takata with his little girl and remained until February 1938. During this time Hayashi made Mrs. Takata a Reiki educator.

Somewhere in the range of 1940 and 1970, Mrs. Takata ran a few Reiki centers and showed numerous classes in Hawaii. In 1973 she showed her five stars in the United States. In December of 1980 Mrs. Takata has passed. Much appreciation and affirmation are perceived for Mrs. Takata in empowering Reiki to spread all through the world. Without her, the arrangement of Reiki may have right up 'til the present stayed obscure but to a chosen few in Japan.

## Dr Usui's Original Reiki Teachings

The most profound otherworldly practices and procedures of the Japanese conventions have stayed behind Japan's shut Reiki society. The first Reiki of Mikao Usui still thrives in Japan yet is impressively unique practically speaking. Outside of Japan there are just three authorized educators of the pre-1922 framework – one of whom is an individual from The Reiki Guild.

# CHAPTER 3
# THE SCIENCE BEHIND REIKI

Reiki is in this manner a type of vitalism – the pre-logical conviction that some profound vitality speeds up the living and is the thing that isolates living things from non-living things. The idea of vitalism was constantly a scholarly placeholder, in charge of whatever parts of science were not as of now comprehended. In any case, as science advanced, in the end we made sense of most of the essential elements of life and there was nothing left for the fundamental power to do. It along these lines blurred from logical reasoning. We can add to that the way that nobody has had the option to give positive proof to the presence of a crucial power – it remains completely obscure to science.

Be that as it may, the subject of science and superstition of the past is the "elective medication" of today. There are some alleged "CAM" modalities that depend on vitalism, including Reiki. Reiki, truth be told, is fundamentally the same as therapeutic contact, another vitality mending methodology that was prevalent among medical caretakers and, despite the fact that it keeps on being utilized, it is substantially less well known. A young lady (Emily Rosa) performed a rich experiment to demonstrate that it was only self-double dealing. Reiki pleasantly moved in to fill the void.

The examination on Reiki and vitality mending when all is said and done, is similar to that of numerous comparative modalities – those with extremely low logical credibility that are not paid attention to by medicinal researchers. The exploration is of low quality, inadequately controlled little examinations that appear to be intended to legitimize Reiki as opposed to check whether it really works. The most as of late distributed investigation, for instance, sees uneasiness levels and self-detailed prosperity in malignancy patient and finds, obviously, that patients feel better when they get the caring consideration of a medical caretaker. The examination is totally uncontrolled and, subsequently, of questionable worth. One should seriously mull over such an examination a total exercise in futility and exertion, as the outcomes were never in uncertainty.

**A 2011 review of Reiki concentrates closed:**

The current research doesn't permit ends in regard to the adequacy or viability of vitality healing. Future examinations ought to cling to existing norms of research on the viability and adequacy of a treatment, and given the mind-boggling character of potential results, cross-disciplinary strategies might be significant. To expand the extent of clinical preliminaries, psychosocial procedures ought to be considered and investigated, instead of rejected as fake treatment

Reiki (articulated raykey) is a type of "vitality healing", basically the Asian version of confidence mending or laying on of hands. Specialists accept they are moving life vitality to the patient, expanding their prosperity. The training is well known among medical caretakers and is polished by attendants at my own foundation (Yale).

Reiki is a Japanese system for stress decrease and unwinding that additionally advances healing. It is managed by "laying on of hands" and depends on the possibility that a concealed "life power vitality" moves through us and is the thing that makes us be alive. And if one's "life power vitality" is low, at that point we are bound to become ill or feel pressure. Assuming it is high, we are progressively fit for being upbeat and sound.

Reiki is in this manner a type of vitalism – the pre-logical conviction that some otherworldly energy vitalizes the living and is the thing that isolates living things from non-living things. The thought of vitalism was constantly a scholarly placeholder, in charge of whatever parts of science were not as of now comprehended. Be that as it may, as science advanced, in the long run we made sense of most of the essential elements of life and there was basically nothing left for the imperative power to do. We can add to that the way that nobody has had the option, to give positive proof to the presence of a crucial power – it remains altogether obscure to science.

Be that as it may, the disposed of science and superstition of the past is the "elective prescription" of today. There are some supposed "CAM" modalities that depend on vitalism, including Reiki. Reiki, truth be told, is fundamentally the same as therapeutic contact, another vitality mending methodology that was well known among medical caretakers, and even though it keeps on being utilized it is significantly less prominent. Emily Rosa performed an exquisite experiment to demonstrate that it was only self-misdirection. Reiki pleasantly moved in to fill the void.

The exploration of Reiki and vitality mending when all is said and done, is like that of numerous comparative modalities – those with exceptionally low logical credibility that are not paid attention to by medicinal researchers. The examination, either of high or low quality, consists in inadequately controlled little investigations that appear to be intended to legitimize Reiki, as opposed to check whether it really works. For instance, they see nervousness levels and self-detailed prosperity in malignant growth and find, obviously, that patients feel better when they get the caring of a medical caretaker. The investigation is totally uncontrolled and of questionable worth. One should seriously mull over such an investigation a total exercise in futility and exertion, as the outcomes were never uncertain.

The current research doesn't allow limitations concerning the viability or adequacy of vitality mending. Future investigations ought to hold fast to existing norms of research on the viability and adequacy of a treatment and given the intricate character of potential results, cross-disciplinary strategies might be important. To expand the extent of clinical preliminaries, psychosocial procedures must be considered and investigated, as opposed to expelled as fake treatment.

As such – existing exploration is a such low quality we can't reach any valuable inference from it. I dissent, notwithstanding, this essentially implies that more research is required. The low believability of utilizing mystical energy that has never been believed to exist by therapeutic science contends something else. Further, the last sentence is odd – it implies the creators are attempting to turn misleading impacts into genuine impacts. This is progressively the technique of elective drug advocates as it turns out to be certain that the vast majority of the modalities they support don't work any better than fake treatment (which means they don't work).

Reiki is present heavily in that field. Distributed at about a similar time as the audit (and in this way excluded in the survey) is a well-planned investigation of Reiki where it was compared with fake Reiki treatment (somebody not prepared in Reiki basically makes an insincere effort) versus normal consideration (no mediation). As anyone might expect, both the genuine Reiki and the hoax Reiki gatherings improved on self-revealed prosperity than the no mediation gathering, yet they were indistinct from one another. In this way Reiki didn't exceed the fake treatment. That implies Reiki doesn't work (at any rate in the normal universe of science-based prescription).

Reiki (articulated raykey) is a type of "vitality healing", basically the Asian adaptation of confidence mending or laying on of hands. Professionals accept they are moving life vitality to the patient, expanding their prosperity. The training is mainstream among medical caretakers and in certainty is polished by attendants at my very own university (Yale).

Reiki is a Japanese system for stress decrease and unwinding that likewise advanced healing. It is controlled by "laying on of hands" and depends on the possibility that a concealed "life power vitality" flows through us and is the thing that makes us alive. Assuming one's "life power vitality" is low, at that point we are bound to become ill or feel pressure and, in case it is high, we are progressively liable for being upbeat and enthusiastic.

Reiki is consequently a type of vitalism – the pre-logical conviction that some otherworldly vitality energizes the being and is the element that isolates living things from non-living things. The thought of vitalis was constantly a scholarly place-holder, in charge of whatever parts of science were not still comprehended. Be that as it may, as science advanced, in the end we made sense of most of the essential elements of life and there was just nothing left for the fundamental power to do. It's in this manner blurred from logical reasoning.

Anyway, the subject of science and superstition of the past is the "elective prescription" of today. There are some alleged "CAM" modalities that depend on vitalism, including Reiki. Reiki, indeed, is fundamentally the same as therapeutic contact, another vitality healing methodology that was prevalent among medical caretakers and in spite of the fact that it keeps on being utilized it is substantially less well known, following the exquisite experiment performed by Emily Rosa to demonstrate that it was only self-duplicity. Reiki pleasantly moved in to fill the void.

The exploration on Reiki and vitality mending when all is said and done, is like that of numerous comparative modalities – those with exceptionally low logical believability that are not paid attention to by restorative researchers. The exploration is of high and low quality, ineffectively controlled little investigations that appear to be intended to legitimize Reiki instead of checking whether it really works. The most as of late distributed examination, for instance, sees tension levels and self-announced prosperity in malignant growth patient and finds, obviously, that patients feel better when they get the thoughtful consideration of an attendant. The examination is totally uncontrolled and in this manner of questionable worth. One should seriously think about such an investigation, a total exercise in futility and exertion, as the outcomes were never uncertain.

The current research doesn't permit ends with respect to the adequacy or viability of vitality mending. Future investigations ought to stick to existing norms of research on the viability and adequacy of a treatment, and given the mind-boggling character of potential results, cross-disciplinary philosophies might be important. To broaden the extent of clinical preliminaries, psychosocial procedures ought to be considered and investigated, instead of expelling them as fake treatment.

As it were – existing examination is at such a such low quality, we can't reach any helpful determination from it. However, this fundamentally implies more research is required. The low credibility of utilizing otherworldly vitality that has never been shown to exist by therapeutic science contends something else. Further, the last sentence is odd – it implies the creators are attempting to turn misleading impacts into genuine impacts. This is progressively the procedure of elective drug advocates as it turns out to be evident that the greater part of the modalities they support don't work any better than fake treatment (which means they don't work).

Reiki is currently unequivocally in that camp. Distributed at about a similar time as the survey (and thusly excluded in the audit), is a well-planned investigation of Reiki where Reiki was contrasted with fake treatment (somebody not prepared in Reiki just makes a cursory effort), versus regular consideration (no mediation). As anyone might expect, both the genuine Reiki and the trick Reiki gatherings improved on self-revealed prosperity more than the no intercession gathering, yet they were undefined from one another. In this way Reiki didn't outrun the treatment. That implies Reiki doesn't work (at any rate in the ordinary universe of science-based prescription).

**The creators finish up:**

The discoveries show that the nearness of an RN giving one-on-one help during chemotherapy was powerful in raising solace and prosperity levels, with or without an endeavored mending vitality field.

I see the creators didn't state that "Reiki doesn't work." This is odd, given that both the treatment and fake treatment gatherings had a similar impact on abstract results. With normal therapeutic mediations we gathered from this result, the treatment doesn't work. Envision a pharmaceutical organization closing:

The discoveries demonstrate that taking a pill during chemotherapy was persuasive in raising solace and prosperity levels, with or without a functioning fixing.

In this manner – taking pills is useful. We should not worry about whether the dynamic fixing has a physiological impact. Reiki supporters seem to have removed a page from the needle therapy handbook. If genuine and hoax needle therapy are both superior to no intervention (they contend), then needle therapy works, regardless of whether genuine or fake treatment.

By demanding that patients must not be treated with fake treatments like Reiki, researchers likewise advocate that they get medications that evidently work better that fake treatment. For example, rub has been proved to improve the prosperity of malignant tumors patients past a misleading impact. Assuming a patient gets a back rub with compassion, time, comprehension and devotion, they would profit by the misleading impact – simply like the

Reiki persistent – at the same time, moreover, they would likely profit from the particular impact of the treatment that back rub does and Reiki doesn't offer.

This is a basic point that I have been making moreover. Basically, you can't legitimize inadequate medication essentially considering this fact, they give a misleading impact. That is on the grounds that viable medications additionally give a similar misleading impact, yet in addition give explicit advantages since they really work.

I would argue that there are additionally numerous potential damages from persuading patients that informal medicines are compelling a result of their vague misleading impacts. This is a duplicity, disregards understanding self-governance and educated assent and sets them up to maybe depend on inadequate "otherworldly" cures for non-self-restricting sicknesses.

All together for doctors and other social insurance experts to suggest a treatment or mending practice to patients, they need proof that it is protected and effective. About security, there have been no detailed negative impacts from Reiki in any of the exploration studies. This is reasonable given that no substance is ingested or connected to the skin and Reiki contact is non-manipulative (and can be offered off the body when required).

## Is Reiki viable?

That leaves the inquiry: is Reiki viable? Or on the other hand, from an analytical point of view, what is Reiki viable for?

A Reiki expert would respond to that question by saying: "Reiki is successful for reestablishing harmony, which can appear in various ways, contingent upon the ebb and flow need of the person." That's not an answer that interests therapeutic analysts, who are used to reading medication for explicit sicknesses instead of medicines to improve health or reestablish harmony.

Regarded restorative research is intended to address quite certain inquiries. Albeit regular drug has since quite a while ago incorporated an idea of homeostasis, or fundamental equalization, there has generally been no unmistakable meaning of this idea that can be utilized to test the theory that Reiki advances balance. Given the unclearness of the term "pressure" and the differences between individuals and the conditions in which they live and work, how might science measure a person's parity?

## What results have been considered?

Until now, the essential results examined in Reiki research have utilized measures for torment, uneasiness and stress, including pulse, circulatory strain, salivary cortisol, just as measures for occupation burnout and minding adequacy. Increasingly explicit measures have been utilized to assess results for stroke recovery, despondency and other ceaseless wellbeing conditions. Given the moderately unpretentious and complex nature of Reiki practice, these measures may not sufficiently catch the lived understanding of those getting Reiki. Measures that join personal satisfaction, quiet fulfillment and stress decrease may have the best potential for showing the advantages of Reiki practice.

## What issues can be encountered when examining Reiki?

Examining modalities, for example, Reiki raises different questions.

## Unsatisfactory quality of randomized controlled preliminaries

The randomized controlled preliminary is appropriate to contemplating the effect of pharmaceutical components (albeit ongoing improvements have demonstrated that even this line of request can be controlled).

In any case, is the straightforwardness of the randomized controlled foundation appropriate to considering treatments that unmistakably inspire complex, multileveled, quick and enduring reactions, for example, seen with Reiki? Many regarded specialists think not and a discourse about how best to examine Reiki and other integrative treatments and mending practices has started. Frameworks hypothesis is progressively observed as giving an increasingly suitable way to deal with concentrating the snare of connections engaged with integrative treatments. Subjective research may likewise give a more extensive focal point in producing important information. An exceptional perplexing variable in Reiki research is controlling for the impact of human touch. Do Reiki beneficiaries have improved results since they have gotten continued human touch? Moreover, how would you make a fake treatment standard for a hands-on mending strategy? In 1999, fake treatment institutionalization was brought into Reiki research, exhibiting that review members couldn't separate between the fake treatment and Reiki. The expansion of a fake treatment branch in Reiki research fortifies investigation structure and addresses the perplexing variable of human touch.

### Powerlessness to archive the biofield

Another obstruction to Reiki research is the powerlessness of contemporary innovation to record the presence of the biofield. Superconducting quantum impedance gadgets (SQUIDs) measure incredibly little attractive fields and may later demonstrate as helpful to this investigation. The speed mechanical advances are being made with may imply that the required innovation is on the very edge of improvement. Nonetheless, it is additionally conceivable that Reiki or biofields lie outside the bioelectromagnetic range. Luckily, it isn't important for science to record the presence of either Reiki or the biofield to gauge the effect of Reiki on the human framework (headache medicine was utilized for a long time before science started to see how it functions). Even if a few impacts of Reiki are quantifiable, for example, improved pulse and circulatory strain, numerous normally detailed advantages of rehashed Reiki sessions (for example, a feeling of profound association and upgraded confidence) may not be quantifiable. It is yet critical to archive these detailed advantages.

Patients who feel more profoundly associated and who just rest easy thinking about themselves are likely easier to treat and better prepared to pursue treatment conventions. Along these lines, Reiki appear to be fundamental, yet in a roundabout way, it might sway therapeutic results by supporting the capacity of patients to get to ordinary prescription and increase an elevated attention to their very own needs.

**What is the status of the research?**

While the discussion on how best to think about integrative treatments, Reiki is picking up steam, research endeavors have been and keep on being made. In any case, investigation into Reiki is simply starting. The National Center for Complementary and Integrative Health

(NCCIH) of the National Institutes of Health (NIH) has finished five investigations taking a look at Reiki's capacity to profit individuals with diabetes, propelled AIDS, prostate disease, fibromyalgia, and stress.

Other distributed investigations have taken a look at the impact of Reiki on proportions of pressure hormones, pulse, and insusceptible responsivity and on emotional reports of anxiety, torment and depression. The investigations to date are normally little and only one out of every odd examination is all around structured. Notwithstanding, covering information from a portion of the more grounded examinations bolsters the capacity of Reiki to decrease uneasiness and torment and proposes its convenience to prompt unwinding, improve weakness and burdensome side effects and fortify general prosperity. The Cochrane Database of Systematic Reviews contains an audit on the utilization of touch treatments (counting Reiki) for torment and a convention for utilization of Reiki for mental side effects.

Reiki has been progressively offered as a component of work environment wellbeing projects to address burnout and improve abilities in medicinal services and different enterprises, too as in college health focuses..

# CHAPTER 4
# THE IMPORTANCE OF INITIATION SIZE

Reiki is an approach to utilize the vitality in your grasp to adjust and revive the existence power vitality inside you. At the point when our life power vitality is high, we are less inclined to become ill. Numerous individuals who have been sick have profited by physical, mental and passionate heling from this hands-on vitality treatment. Through Reiki attunements, you can figure out how to take advantage of the existent power vitality and renew and mend yourself as well as other people. For some, the attunement or commencement procedure begins in 1st Degree Reiki Practitioners Healing Training. For other people, it is the formal commencement into mending others performed at the Reiki ace level. This book examines the job of attunement in Levels 1, 2 and Masters Reiki preparing.

With numerous reports in the media about vitality mending, more individuals are interested and looking for an introduction to vitality recuperating. Standard Reiki attunements is a demonstrated method to guarantee long haul great health. One of the attractions of Reiki is that anybody can figure out how to utilize it. Reiki bosses mend by widespread vitality or Qi, through the palms. This life renewing vitality practice is passed on from ace to student.

Reiki doesn't just treat physical wellbeing yet in addition enthusiastic, mental and otherworldly health. Ensuring your life power vitality is adjusted is the most ideal approach to guarantee all-encompassing wellbeing. This Japanese healing strategy is progressively being utilized by Western countries as a component of the mending process. Thus, request is expanding for prepared experts who can perform Reiki attunements.

## Solution to choosing Reiki Initiation Master

Picking the privilege of a Reiki expert is essential to the achievement of your attunements in every one of the three degrees of training. Since Mikao Usui created Reiki in 1922, numerous varieties have pursued. Request that your planned educator clarifies their preparation and experience utilizing Reiki. Ask them to discuss their way of thinking and how it might contrast from that of other Reiki masters. And critically, get some information about any progressions or upgrades to their Reiki program from the customary practice.

The International Center for Reiki, for instance, underlines the convention of the customary Tibetan methods as well as the Usui Reiki techniques. This program affirms to make changes in accordance with the first Reiki technique. Truth be told, there are a few ancestries of Reiki instructed in Japan today – some of them hidden and others vigorously impacted by the Western procedures. Guarantee you comprehend the Reiki procedure being offered. Specifically inquire as to why this framework is the best for you.

Functional contemplations incorporate booking. When is the class held and for how long? Weekend courses have turned out to be well known however would a weeklong retreat be better for you? Charges shift extraordinarily today among schools. To teach Reiki to other people, every one of the three levels is required. At the ace level, you will be initiated into healing others. Consider at the time, cash and different assets you will require to finish Reiki master's level.

Reiki is more physically private than many specialist understanding relationships. Ask yourself how agreeable you would lie on a table for an hour getting Reiki medication from your educator. Reiki includes opening yourself up profoundly and emotionally. If you wind up guarded or bashful, keep on talking to Reiki teachers. Assess your mood. Do you feel upbeat around this person? Does the educator make you like yourself?

## Planning for the Initiation Process

Clear your calendar of all commitments. If you have a ton of work and family worry during your Reiki class, it will be more sincere to open yourself up to the vitality procedure. Try not to plan any significant get-togethers during your Reiki commencement forms, particularly those including liquor.

Sanitize your arrangement of substances. Take out caffeine, liquor, meat and sugar from your diet. Consider fasting for a couple of days.

Meditate for an hour every day. This is a significant advance that will enable you to quiet your psyche and manage your vitality stream before the exercises start. You will get more from Reiki preparing Assuming you are now raising your vitality vibrations.

Attempt and maintain a strategic distance from unpleasant circumstances and individuals. Once more, this is to help guarantee a quiet, thoughtful attitude.

Invest more energy among nature. Another unwinding strategy is to take a stroll on a bright day. Take a walk around the recreation center or by the sea as opposed to staring at the TV.

# The Reiki Attunement Process

## What is Reiki Initiation?

Ace Usui got his capacity to take advantage of Reiki vitality through an otherworldly reflection. The custom of passing Reiki down from ace to understudy proceeds. Attunement is another term for Initiation, or "reiju" in Japanese. Pamela Miles, a Reiki specialist, makes a noteworthy distinction between the terms "attunement" and "inception" on her blog. Understanding the genuine significance of inception will extend your Reiki practice. Quickly, attunement is frequently characterized as the strict exchange of all-inclusive vitality from master to understudy, supplying the understudy with the capacity to turn into a healer. Though inception alludes to the start of learning discipline. Learning, as Miles notes, includes posing inquiries can be constant. Like the nonstop renewal of vitality, the professional ought to constantly build up their abilities as a vitality healer. While inception better catches the genuine plan of Reiki healing, we will keep on utilizing the famous term "attunement" here. Yet rather than considering attunement a privilege of entry as a vitality healer, attempt and think about every attunement procedure as the start of a constant learning process.

Reiki Attunement - An approach Through the Three Reiki Levels

The attunement or commencement procedure happens in every one of the three degrees of Reiki: Reiki 1, Reiki 2 and Master level. At each level the Master initiates the student with more grounded mending vitality as they move to more elevated amounts of vitality vibration.

Reiki 1 includes four commencements of the physical body. To become an affirmed level 1 Reiki expert, you will find out about the vitality meridians of the body, the Reiki hand positions and Reiki life systems; and at last how to utilize the Reiki vitality framework to heal yourself as well as other people. When this learning is effectively aced, the Level 1 Reiki attunement must be given by a Certified Reiki Master. The function often takes 20 or 30 minutes.

Reiki 2 starts the unpretentious or air body. Three Reiki images are taught – control, mental and separation. Notwithstanding the sacrosanct symbols, 2ndDegree Certified Reiki Practitioners Training teach extra images and hand positions. A few courses will likewise show removed Reiki remedy at this stage.

The Reiki Master level initiates the understudy into instructing Reiki. The Master image is educated. A few Masters allude to this third from as the official attunement or inception form as a vitality healer. At Level 3, you will figure out how to perform Reiki attunement on others.

## Separation Reiki Attunement

Numerous individuals offer the chance to get Reiki and different types of vitality mending at a distance. While some separation healers have demonstrated that they draw from an amazing vitality source, most Reiki experts don't prescribe separation mending. Episodically, many people from those utilizing separation recuperating report that the vitality isn't as solid. A few masters accept that the physical touch is basic to convey the required mending vitality. Handy contemplations incorporate challenges getting neighborhood references and joining nearby Reiki gatherings where your healer likewise has a place. In the case of preparing in Reiki or looking for mending, similar capabilities for picking a Reiki ace must be utilized.

## The Reiki Ideals

Learning the Reiki procedures and going through all phases of attunement/inception is just a piece of the road toward turning into a mindful vitality healer. You should likewise maintain the good and moral norms of a Reiki vitality healers. The Reiki Ideals were created by Reiki organizer Usui Mikao. The Reiki Ideals guarantee the sound and dependable routine with regards to Reiki. They are an attestation that you are the healer and in charge of your own demonstrations of mending. The first Reiki beliefs are the following:

· The mystery specialty of welcoming bliss.

· The marvelous medication of everything being equal.

· Only for now, don't outrage.

· Try not to stress and be loaded up with appreciation.

· Dedicate yourself to your work. Be thoughtful to individuals.

· Each morning and night join your hands in prayer.

· Ask these words to your heart.

· Furthermore, serenade these words with your mouth.

**Check out Usui Reiki Treatment for the improvement of body and psyche**

When you have learned Reiki, the capacity to mend yourself as well as other people physically, rationally, sincerely and profoundly lasts for a lifetime. Like any learning, assuming you seek after nonstop learning – that is, continually addressing and finding out more – your Reiki mending vitality will stay solid and even more, profoundly receptive to the general vitality source. While healing others is a steady wellspring of reconnection with the vitality source, getting attunements now and again from different bosses will keep you finely sensitive to the vitality source.

## Inception or attunement?

Sometime after the demise of Hawayo Takata in December 1980, "attunement" started springing up. Numerous Reiki experts presently use it only for the procedure Mrs. Takata alluded to as inception ("reiju" in Japanese).

Be sure that the inception procedure is baffling, "commencement" is entirely clear. It alludes to starting.

Inception is the procedure by which a master offers a student the capacity to rehearse. Commencement ancestry keeps the training alive and is regular in Asian profound procedures.

The procedure of inception is innately baffling; what it achieves — empowering us to rehearse — isn't.

Similarly, as the pith of training is to start once more, commencement can be rehashed. Usui offered reiju to his students each time they gathered to rehearse.

The ascent of "attunement" appears to have put a conclusion to addressing. It urged specialists to see Reiki as a specific vibration of "vitality" to which individuals should be "adjusted" to rehearse. This disarray — that one is receptive to vitality as opposed to started into training — has taken on its very own existence and is currently for the most part introduced as certainty.

In any case, it is anything but a reality. It's a conviction. What's more, if Reiki practice is predicated on conviction, it's never again a training; it turns into a religion.

When you notice it that way — which is how individuals outside the New Age people group will, in general, notice it — is it so astonishing that some religious societies are against Reiki practice?

## Demystifying inception, in a manner of speaking

It's difficult to really demystify inception. Considering this fact, the procedure itself is supernatural. In any case, while the inception procedure is baffling, what it achieves is down to earth and normally unmistakable. Individuals who get a Reiki inception might possibly see something during the procedure of commencement, however I would say, they see the impact.

As a youthful Reiki ace, I committed the error maybe all new masters make: I blabbered.

After some time, I realized that my mission isn't to clarify Reiki. Or maybe, my duty as a Reiki ace is just to show understudies how to rehearse Reiki, to get them to rehearse day by day self-treatment and to give them the certainty that they really can rehearse effectively.

## Is inception enough?

I realize every one of my student's needs is the inception; I, likewise, realize they don't have the foggiest idea about that. I can't anticipate that they should trust me, nor do I need them to. I need understudies to build up their very own certainty. What's more, nothing I state can make certainty the path in-class practice does.

In my First-degree classes, we move into the first of the four inceptions offered in Hawayo Takata's genealogy directly after the welcome and presentations. I, at that point, lead the understudies through their first altered Reiki self-practice. After this short introductory practice and before they open their eyes, I request that they see any little contrast between the way they feel currently contrasted with how they felt when they began.

When I've delicately driven them out of their training session, the understudies share what they saw during their first practice. I don't recall the last time somebody didn't see anything.

In any event, individuals feel more settled, increasingly focused, progressively loose — and that is not how they expected to feel sitting discreetly in a gathering of outsiders.

The procedure of commencement is innately secretive; what it achieves — empowering us to rehearse — isn't.

Reiki Initiations are here to push you to reconnect with your picked life way and to turn into a channel for this Universal Life Healing Energy. It is the establishment for your own healing in your life and a chance to pass it onto other living creatures in the hour of this major vivacious progress from the third dimensional Energy to the fifth dimensional Energy. It is a mending practice and a method for living with profound regard, sympathy and empathy for the Soul and each living being including yourself, other individuals, creatures, plants and Mother Earth.

Reiki Initiations can raise your cognizance to a more prominent level and bring understanding of your actual way and subsequently the motivation to your own picked educational experience, the significance (or certainty) of disease or a problem and learning involved. Through Reiki

Initiations your own vitality is being raised, your levels of awareness and mindfulness start developing – so significant from now on, to stay aware of this approaching high fifth dimensional Energy.

## SO, DO WE NEED INITIATION TO BE ABLE TO USE REIKI?

Indeed, we should be initiated by a Reiki Master Teacher, who has accurately adjusted themselves. Reiki is a high, sacred Life Healing Energy and to have the option to arrive at that level our energy and awareness should be raised. We cannot do this by ourselves, a Reiki Master should be there for us to take us through those stages. This is the way Master Usui taught his understudies. There is a significant minute in each person's life when we believe we are reconnecting with our actual self and the Holy Source that individuals call Mother/Father God.

In contrast to other recuperating expressions, Reiki is passed from ace to understudy through a Reiki attunement that allows the understudy to interfere with the all-inclusive Reiki source.

### So, what is Involved for Each Reiki Attunement?

Be aware that in a Reiki level 1 attunement, students are receptive to three unique images, each speaking to an alternate part of Reiki vitality: control, mental/passionate equalization and separation healing. Every understudy gets attunements to these 3 images in four separate occasions and with every reiteration the association develops.

Therefore, the attunements for Reiki level 2 and Reiki ace are comparative in nature, yet include various images, each with an alternate importance to opening your vivacious pathways.

### What feeling comes through Attunement?

Be aware that getting a Reiki attunement is a ground-breaking, profound experience, as your lively pathways are opened by a Reiki ace. This vivacious opening permits the Reiki vitality to stream uninhibitedly through your body to affect your wellbeing and the soundness of others.

The sentiment of a Reiki attunement is an individual one, yet understudies regularly report that they feel an energy through their body and shivering from their head to their toes as the Reiki vitality pathways are opened.

The opening of an attunement has the impact of enhancing other lively mending and directing pathways and understudies report that accepting an attunement causes expanded instinctive mindfulness and improves any intrinsic clairvoyant affectability.

## How Do You Prepare for an Attunement?

Meanwhile, how you get ready for a Reiki attunement relies upon your very own profound practice. Opening a vigorous pathway is no light issue and keeping in mind that it's important to do anything so as to get ready to get a Reiki attunement, most understudies decide to reconnect with their own otherworldly practice before their attunement, to increase the general impacts of the attunement and amplify its transformative power.

One prescribed arrangement for planning for a Reiki attunement involves a 3-day rinse before your attunement. Abstain from eating overwhelming nourishments, limit or dispose of caffeine, sugar, tobacco or liquor. Invest your energy perusing or pondering instead of sitting in front of the TV. Endeavor to discharge negative feelings, for example outrage or desire.

These arrangements will enable you to be increasingly prepared to acknowledge the otherworldly change and urge the attunement to have significant, long haul impacts on your life and prosperity.

## Does an Attunement Need to be Renewed?

When you have been sensitive to Reiki, the Reiki vitality will course through you for an incredible remainder. Your capacity to channel and move Reiki vitality stays with you, as the endowment of Reiki tails you and encourages you for an incredible remainder.

**So, what Are the Benefits of Receiving Attunements Remotely?**

In-person classes are regularly instructed rapidly, without much time for understudies to consolidate the data. The attunements are given as one huge mob toward the part of the arrangement, without time for the understudies to plan for the significant otherworldly change that an attunement involves. By studying remotely, you can learn and incorporate the advantages of Reiki at your own pace and take a couple of days to set yourself up for your attunement before you get it.

Reiki is a thrilling practice and a great part of the Reiki you get and convey all through a mind-blowing remainder will be a long time experience. Starting your Reiki venture remotely encourages you to get ready for an existence of Reiki without outskirts.

# CHAPTER 5
# STANDARDS OF REIKI

The genuine Reiki standards are at the very heart of the first Reiki lessons. They are given a great deal of room on the dedication stone and it is recommended that they're rehashed each day. Thusly, you may discover what I, in the long run, found for myself: they are totally, absolutely accommodating. I can't go without them anymore. I would venture to express that they have changed my life.

This is an interpretation of the first form from the commemoration stone:

· Only for now,

· Try not to be irate.

· Try not to stress.

· Be thankful.

· Do your work with industriousness.

· Be benevolent to other people.

· Rehash, rehash, rehash

In the Japanese perception, the standards are viewed as a vital aspect for opening to Reiki. Mikao Usui alluded to them as 'the mystery strategy to welcome bliss' and the 'extraordinary prescription to fix all diseases'. He requested that his students sit in Gassho and rehash them each morning and each night.

Use auto-entrancing. Let's assume them, think them, dream them. Become them.

The Reiki standards are devices to prepare the psyche. They add a component of brain science to Reiki and work on cognizant and subliminal levels.

It is anything but difficult to fill a whole book with the numerous layers of the standards, however for the present I will simply focus on a couple of key perspectives. You will discover more by applying them.

Mother Teresa had a breathtaking hands-on methodology: 'We have just today. Allow us to start.' This is the thing that this prologue to the standards urges us to do: start. Actualize the standards. Try not to pause!

Having an opportunity or not, involves decision. 'Only for now' additionally signifies: 'I may have attempted yesterday, I might not have consistently succeeded yesterday, yet yesterday is no more. Today is one more day, another possibility and I will attempt once more. Over and over, until I succeed.' For the greater part of us, stress is a noteworthy issue in our day by day lives. Assuming only for one day we could attempt to quit stressing so much, we could all live more gently which thus, will likewise carry harmony to other people. Not to mention, lowering your pressure will likewise profit your wellbeing! So only for now trust the Spirit, Source, God (or yourself!) and realize that everything is turning out fine and dandy. It generally does.

When I talk about this standard on a Reiki course, the response isn't constantly positive. We appear to be enormously impervious to either tolerating or going up against displeasure. Many individuals have proposed rephrasing the rule. They would want to repeat 'I am quiet' or 'I am calm' or 'I am loose.' If an average morning for you includes being cut off by another driver on your way to work, you most likely will be outraged. Why not simply take a full breath, unwind, pardon and let it go? What will you accomplish by staying furious and slicing him off to "settle the score with him?" Nothing. All that you'll wind up with is a raised pulse (and more pressure!) which isn't useful for your prosperity.

Basically rehashing 'Don't be furious' can make us feel awkward. The negative stating raises outrage as opposed to stifling it. Yet, that is what it is intended to do. This standard isn't a certification. It isn't intended to artificially glamorize, stifle or discredit outrage – it's intended to bring it up. So, to manage it, we should know about it.

In the wake of rehashing 'Don't be irate' a couple of times, an understudy of mine once begun crying. Recollections of a gigantic showdown with her mom flashed up – from 15 years prior! She was stunned to find that this episode was still so instilled in her psyche that a straightforward exercise could bring it up. Be that as it may, Reiki had at last carried her the solidarity to manage it.

Harboring outrage is rarely advantageous, either for the individual clutching (it makes us both hopeless and sick) or for the individual that is in the long run coordinated. The Buddha closed: 'You won't be rebuffed for your resentment; you will be rebuffed by your outrage.'

The guideline doesn't state: 'Handle your indignation.' Nor: 'Offer your outrage.' It says: 'Don't be irate.' Which signifies: 'Be something different.' It advises us that we have the power to decide.

Outrage is activated by disillusionment, stun, weakness – or simply being intruded. We were anticipating something that ended up being extraordinary. So, what happens at that point?

The synthetic concoctions that are along these lines discharged and that make us 'feel' outrage are managed by the body rapidly. They are totally flushed out of our framework in under 90 seconds. All we need do is take a full breath and hang on for a moment – and our reaction to the circumstance shouldn't be coordinated by indignation, yet by whatever we supplant it with. We are continually requesting more and just observing what we don't have. We should pursue one day to be thankful for what we do have — like a vocation, a vehicle that takes you where you have to go, a rooftop over your head, great wellbeing and a family that cherishes you genuinely and underpins you. Be aware that when we are thankful for what we have, we will attract greatness. The law of fascination expresses that like draws in like and need pulls in need, so remain positive and be appreciative for what you have.

Would we be able to change the circumstances? Would we be able to change our demeanor? Learn for next time? Acknowledge? Excuse? Or then again, perhaps, make a move? Does our annoyance lead us to improve the world a spot? Presently outrage transforms into something valuable: an instrument for change. What's more, there's no compelling reason to clutch it. This Reiki rule offers the chance to respond in an unexpected way.

## Try not to stress

During the years between my insolvency and my disclosure of Reiki, a companion once inquired as to whether I had a wish for the New Year. I stated: 'To get up one morning unafraid.' So, for me to expound on 'Don't stress' resembles being a burglar publicizing criminal alerts. Be that as it may, a recuperating one. Reiki slowly brought assistance. Also, with it trust.

Stress is only absence of trust: 'Last time something troublesome occurred, so it may happen again tomorrow.' Well, it may. Or then again it may not. If it does, we must manage it. Tomorrow. Not today. Assuming it doesn't, our stress will have been a finished exercise in futility. I'm certain I squandered long stretches of my life stressing.

Assuming stress leads to appropriate arrangement, it has filled its need. We can release it and leave the rest to the universe. What's more, we can send Reiki to the issue. So, it's more difficult than one might expect, obviously. Everybody experiences troublesome stages and some of the time they appear to keep going forever. However, they don't. One day they will have passed.

So, the more we let go of our stresses, the more we open to synchronicity. Also, marvels.

## Be appreciative

Some time back this standard was the theme of a Reiki Share – and we did a down to earth practice as well. Each member was approached to record five things they were thankful for. Some began composition straight away, some paused for a minute to do an internal pursuit, yet a while later nearly everybody grumbled that five weren't enough – they'd found many people from something else!

The great old appreciation rundown is a splendid apparatus to make us mindful that there are things we're thankful for. We simply tend to coolly disregard (the well-known glass-half-empty frame of mind).

When we understand we are appreciative, we can frequently feel a practically physical sensation in our entire body. Our vitality turns into the glad vibration of appreciation.

An understudy referenced that while giving a Reiki treatment once, she was overpowered by appreciation for the association. When this came in, the warmth in her grasp significantly increased. Thankfulness is an extraordinary device for clearing blockages.

## Do your work with persistence

When I initially heard this guideline, it sounded odd. What is otherworldly about concentrating on your work? It took some time before it occurred to me that it wasn't just about work, it was about as long as we can remember. Doing your work genuinely brings more meaning into your life. When you do your work genuinely and with reason, by the day's end you'll like yourself and be increasingly satisfied about your work.

Whatever we do, whatever circumstance we are in, we must act with steadiness. In contemporary language, this implies we must assume liability for our life. Where we are may not be our decision, yet how we act unquestionably is.

We are never in an inappropriate spot, truth be told: we are in the place the Universe set us. Regardless of whether we know it or not, we are here for a reason. We can take advantage of it if we apply three essential thoughts. Care. Regard. Trustworthiness.

However, this boils down to having a shave in the first part of the day (today I mined in a surge and as of now sport somewhat cut), to tune in to the individual we are having a discussion with (my sister lately saw that I wasn't giving her my full focus on the telephone) and to doing our activity. Fundamentally, every undertaking will improve if we do it with steadiness.

What's more, obviously, the steadier we are with Reiki itself, the more it can transform us.

## Be benevolent to other people

I once participated in an activity at a profound class. Combined up with someone we barely knew, or even a total outsider, we were approached to give them a compliment. First, there was a snapshot of quietness – the majority of us didn't know what to do. At that point individuals started to 'decidedly analyze' their accomplice. The principal individual turned out with: "Cool shoes." Then it was: "Decent glasses" and "You have delightful eyes". "Do you realize that you have an astounding smile?", "I appreciate your fearlessness, going to this seminar all alone." A couple of minutes later, the room was loaded up with cheerful individuals. The whole vitality had changed. What you give out, you get back ten times. Be pleasant, adoring and minding to everybody, regardless of whether it's not your favorite individual on the planet. We deserve love and thoughtfulness. Toward the day's end we will rest easy thinking about ourselves for bringing some light and love into another person's day, regardless of whether it's only for a minute.

Despite the fact that it may appear to be somewhat overpowering to live by each of the five of this standards every day, you can begin today with the difficult only one. You will be significantly more joyful by the end of the day, I guarantee.

Benevolence doesn't need to be troublesome. It very well may offer your extra room to a companion (as transpired when I lost my home – thank you, Ari and Bob!); it very well may offer a grin to the clerk in the store. Furthermore, obviously Reiki is a stunning device for sharing graciousness.

## Exercise: Reciting the standards

I would unequivocally prescribe following Mikao Usui's recommendation. Each morning and each night sit for a minute in Gassho and rehash the standards.

In any case, if it's not too much trouble take as much time as necessary. I sometimes stop abruptly and figure: You didn't mean it that way! What's more, start once more: 'Only for now, I won't be irate [then I take a brief reprieve and check whether I'm holding outrage or sentiments of resentment], I won't stress [pause once more: Am I stressing? Have I given my stresses over to Reiki?], I will be appreciative [pause again to perceive what comes up], I will do my work with constancy [where do I have to improve?] and I will be caring to others [anyone specifically today?].'

# DIFFERENT PRINCIPLES YOU SHOULD CONSIDER

## Inviting Happiness: The Secret Art Involved

It has been a very long time since these standards were first advised in my Reiki 1 class and keeping in mind that I worked with these standards right off the bat, my own work with them has turned out to be less so in the years that followed. Hatsurei-Ho resuscitated that enthusiasm for the standards just as giving me a preface to the rules that put into setting what I wasn't educated in my Reiki 1 class; "The mystery craft of welcoming bliss; the otherworldly drug for all infections is this".

## By adding Power to the Principles mentioned

What could understand about the 5 Principles were two things. First, if the comprehension from trance specialists and self-improvement pioneers is valid, that our intuitive personality doesn't perceive "not". At that point for what reason are the 5 Reiki Principles utilize expressions as "Don't get angry", "Don't worry"? In deduction, progressively about this stating, it appeared to turn out to be less and less self-enabling as I discussed it. Yet, I've been encouraging my understudies for a while now about how utilizing the 5 Principles can prompt self-development and more noteworthy individual empowerment. Therefore, I gathered that there must be an approach to add capacity to these standards.

Second, and with all due regard to Master Usui, if there is an approach to alter the wording of the standards to help make a more noteworthy self-strength for myself and my understudies, would I be able to build up a bit by bit process that joins the 5 Principles that will encourage this development?

For as far back as months, I've been practicing Hatsurei-Ho, a Japanese Reiki contemplation procedure which fuses the presenting of the 5 Reiki Principles. What struck me half a month into this training was the inclination I got from the 5 Principles; that a "stern somebody" was remaining over me instructing me about what not to do.

**New Phrasing for the Five Reiki Principles**

What introduced itself was a new stating for the 5 Reiki Principles and a procedure for utilizing this new wording any Reiki or non-Reiki-prepared professional can use for self-change.

Become acquainted with the Reiki Principles.

The altered standards are as per the following.

Only for Today:

*I discharge furious musings and sentiments*

*I discharge considerations of stress*

*I'm thankful for my numerous gifts*

*I work on extending my cognizance*

*I'm delicate with all creatures including myself.*

These words mean to me it is my decision to do these things or not. When I speak them, I get myself quieter and more enabled to make my life as I choose. What this new stating brought is a procedure for utilizing every one of the standards deliberately to inspire inner growth. Here is the procedure.

**The most effective method to utilize the 5 Principles for Personal Growth**

1) After you introduce the preface ("The mystery craft of welcoming joy; the profound prescription for all infections is this") think or state so anyone can hear: "Only for Today, I discharge furious contemplations and sentiments."

2) Think about the occasions of that day (or in case you're doing this in the first part of the day, the earlier day) when you lost control and check whether you can perceive that outrage lives inside you, it isn't derived from the outside. The resentment you felt was activated by an event

not depending on you, however the occasion wouldn't have emotionally affected you if you didn't have that irate vitality inside you.

Presently, return in your memory to the last couple of times you responded to something with displeasure (or assuming you can, discover an occasion from your past that appears to be indistinguishable from the present, one that raised your annoyance) and check whether there are any similarities to your current irate contemplations and feelings. Now, ask your (Reiki) guides, higher self, holy messengers and masters from light and love to enable you to let this furious vitality you are holding from the past go. Ask these profound aides to change this furious vitality once more, which is the most astounding healing. Take 1-2 profound, slow breaths and on each breathe out, discharge any staying overwhelming inclination vitality from your physical body.

3) Next, do the same thing with the second standard "Only For Today, I discharge musings of worry". Think about the occasions of that day (or in case you're doing this toward the beginning of the day, the earlier day) when you felt stressed and check whether you can perceive that stress lives inside you, if it isn't originating from worries about some future event that hasn't occurred yet. The stress you felt was activated by contemplating some future occasion outside of you, however the occasion itself wouldn't have

emotionally affected you assuming you didn't have that negative energy. Now, return in your memory to the last couple of times you responded to something with stress (or if you can, think about an occasion from your past that appears to be indistinguishable from the present one that raised your stress) and check whether there are any similitudes to your current considerations and sentiments of worry. Ask your (Reiki) aides, blessed messengers and experts to enable you to let the vitality of stress (and the considerations that triggered it) go now. Request that these profound assistants change this stress vitality once again into positive energy. Take 1-2 profound, slow breaths and on each breathe out, discharge any staying substantial inclination vitality from your physical body and aura. When you are finished with musings of stress, go onto the third guideline.

4) Think or state so anyone can hear: "Only for Today, I'm appreciative for my numerous blessings". Name, picture and feel thankful for each gift (individual, object, circumstance) in your life. Let your heart extend as you do so. Take some time with this. When you are finished with this procedure, go onto the fourth standard.

5) Think or state the fourth standard for all to hear: "Only For Today, I work on extending my awareness" and imagine or recognize every situation of that day or the earlier day where you tried to grow your cognizance

(working with the 5 Principles, pondering, seeing somebody's conduct in another light, feeling appreciative, doing an unwinding exercise and so forth).

6) Think or state the fifth rule so anyone can hear: "Only for Today, I'm delicate with all creatures including myself" and recall times that day or the past one when you were or weren't delicate with others or yourself. Replay them in your brain and ask your (Reiki) aides, holy messengers and bosses from light and love to enable you to release any sentiments of blame or nervousness now. Ask these profound assistants to change this vitality once again into the most elevated mending and development for all. Take 1-2 profound, slow breaths and on each breathe out, discharge any staying overwhelming energy from your physical body.

## A Work in Progress

This technique for utilizing the standards is a work in progress and some of you may be already accomplishing something similar. For the individuals who are discovering this data and strategy now, I trust you'll try it out and see for yourselves (and your understudies) what we find as we keep on utilizing the endowment of Reiki to make more prominent parity and harmony inside ourselves and, by augmentation, the world.

## THE REIKI SYMBOLS

Reiki symbols are utilized in the training of Usui Reiki, an elective type of healing born about 100 years back in Japan by Mikao Usui. The word "Reiki" comes from two Japanese words: "rei" and "ki". "Rei" signifies "higher power" or "otherworldly control." "Ki" signifies "vitality." Put together, Reiki can be inexactly interpreted as "spiritual life power vitality."

Reiki healers practice attunement (some of the time called inception) by moving their hands over the body along the lines of the five customary images. These signals control the progression of all-inclusive vitality called ki (or qi) through the body with the objective of advancing physical or mental healing.

A common Reiki session takes somewhere between 60 minutes and an hour and a half and customers are approached either by resting on a back-rub table or seated. Individuals can remain completely dressed during the Reiki session and direct physical contact is uncommon. Professionals ordinarily start working either at a patient's head or feet, moving gradually along the body as they control their ki.

Reiki images don't hold any extraordinary power themselves. They were formulated as showing devices for

Reiki understudies. It is the objective of the specialist's center that stimulates these images. The accompanying five Reiki images are considered the most sacred. Each might be alluded to by its Japanese name or by its expectation, a representative name that speaks to its motivations in the training.

Reiki is a profoundly guided life power vitality utilized as a non-physical recuperating practice. Created by Mikao Usui, Reiki isn't a religion nor is it taught in the standard form – rather it is transmitted from the ace to the understudy during an "attunement." But don't get too excited for now – there's still plenty to think about.

## Reiki with Intention

While to turn into a Reiki ace one should live in a manner that advances concordance, Reiki isn't subject to one's scholarly limit or profound improvement. You don't need to believe in Reiki with for it to work.

## Five Reiki Symbols to Open Your Mind

To help with this agreeable development, five Reiki images were created as showing devices for understudies and are intended to be keys that open the entryway to a higher personality. These images may appear to be baffling and to some degree threatening from the start, yet they are extremely simple to get a handle on. The Reiki images depend on the Japanese composition framework, Kanji, and ought to be drawn or envisioned as instructed during the Reiki 2 Attunement. By envisioning these images, the client is immediately associated with the general life power and every negative inclination is abrogated.

In the old Reiki tradition, it was accepted that these images are sacred and must be revealed uniquely to the individuals who are started at the Reiki 2 level. As Reiki turns out to be progressively famous and across the board, there are different varieties of these images. Be that as it may, this is cause for little worry as the genuine power in Reiki images lies in their goal.

Here are the five Reiki images that will help you understand whether you're prepared to take your profound voyage to the following level.

### The Power Reiki Symbol

Japanese Name: Cho Ku Rei
Intention: Light Switch
Purposes: Manifestation, increased power, quickened mending, recuperating impetus, insurance

Cho Ku Rei, or the power image, for the most part signifies "Spot the intensity of the universe here". This image can be utilized whenever during a treatment, yet is particularly successful toward the start or part of the arrangement. It is frequently identified with a light switch as it will probably, in a flash, support your capacities.

The curl like structure of this image is inconceivably telling. The loop can grow and contract to direct the "ki" energies and can likewise be utilized as a pipe of sorts to increase and center power or to diminish and discharge vitality when utilized backwards. The loop can likewise be utilized to close a space around the recipient or a zone to shut out negative energies and to keep energies got from leaving. The power symbol, cho ku rei, is used to increment or lessen power (contingent upon the heading in which it is drawn).

Its aim is the light switch, speaking to its capacity to enlighten or illuminate profoundly. Its recognizing image is a loop, which Reiki experts accept as the controller of qi, extending and contracting as the vitality streams all through the body. Power comes in various structures with cho ku rei. It might be utilized as an impetus for physical healing, purging or sanitization. It might likewise be utilized to concentrate.

## The Mental and Emotional Reiki Symbol

Japanese Name: Sei Hei Ki
Intention: Balance
Purposes: Improved memory, emotional healing, mental balance


Otherwise called the Harmony symbol, Sei Hei Ki (articulated "State Hay-Key") unites the cerebrum and the body. By and large, it means "God and man become one,". Sei Hei Ki discharges profound established mental antagonism from the body into the Universe. Making this image your partner is a venture that will reimburse you through an amazing span. Sei Hei Ki is "faithful companion," particularly at whatever point you are confronting challenges. The Sei Hei Ki symbolizes concordance. Its expectation is purification and it is utilized for mental and enthusiastic mending. The image looks like a wave washing over a shoreline or the wing of a fledgling in flight and it is drawn with a general motion. Experts may utilize this expectation during medication for sorrow to reestablish the body's otherworldly harmony. It might likewise be utilized to help individuals recuperate from past physical or psychical injury or to unblock inventive energies.

## The Connection Reiki Symbol

Japanese Name: Hon Sha Ze Sho Nen
Intention: Timelessness
Purposes: Distant mending, past/present/future, recuperating karma, profound association

Otherwise called the "Separation Symbol," Hon Sha Ze Sho Nen (articulated "Hon-Sha-Zee-Show-Nen") signifies "No past, no present, no future" and is to broaden controls and send Reiki energies over a long separation. It symbolizes a shape shifter that can sneak past reality. In any case, don't concentrate its endeavors on a particular issue – rather you should send its Energies Without Limitations and they will go where they are required. Hon Sha Ze Sho Nen additionally offers access to the "Akashic Records" or the existence records of the spirit. Along these lines, be aware that it very well may be utilized to dissipate injury from previous existence encounters for profound karmic healing. Hon Sha Ze Sho Nen is utilized when sending qi crosswise over long distances. Its goal is agelessness and it is here and there called pagoda for the pinnacle like appearance of the characters when worked out. In medications, the aim is accustomed to uniting individuals crosswise over existence. Hon Sha Ze Sho Nen can likewise change itself into a key that will open the Akashic records, which a few specialists accept to be a wellspring of all human awareness. It is a basic apparatus for the Reiki practitioner working on internal identity or previous existence issues with customers.

## The Master Reiki Symbol

Japanese Name: Dai Ko Myo
Intention: Enlightenment
Purposes: Empowerment, soul mending, unity


One of the most dominant images, Dai Ko Myo is just to be utilized by Reiki Masters as it consolidates the intensity of the initial three images, Cho Ku Rei, Sei He Ki and Hon Sha Ze Sho Nen. The image for the most part signifies "Incredible Enlightenment" or "Splendid Shining Light." It speaks to all that is Reiki and is accepted to be the core of Reiki. Although only here and there utilized for explicit reasons, this image rather improves the recuperating impacts of each type of Reiki and fills in as an update that Reiki is love and accessible to everybody. Dai Ko Myo, the ace image, speaks to all that is Reiki. Its goal is edification. The image is utilized by Reiki experts just when adjusting starts. The image recuperates the healers by joining the intensity of the congruity, power and separation images. It is the most mind boggling of the images to draw with the hand during a Reiki session.


## Full Concept on Reiki Symbol

Japanese Name: Raku
Intention: Grounding
Purposes: Kundalini Healing, hara connection, chakra alignment

The Raku image is the last image learned by Usui Reiki Masters and is utilized exclusively during the last phase of the Reiki attunement procedure to seal vitality into the seven chakras. Its will likely ground and seal the recently stirred Reiki energies. Otherwise called the "Fire Serpent," the striking lightning jolt image is drawn downwards from the sky to the earth and speaks to the life-power vitality that keeps running down the spine, through our chakras. The causes of this image are less clear as it was not initially educated by Usui. Rather, it is guessed that Raku is an antiquated Tibetan recuperating specialty of self-dominance and brought toward the west by Arthur Robertson, an understudy of Reiki Master Iris Ishikuro. The Raku symbol is utilized during the last phase of the Reiki attunement process. Its goal is stabilizing. Specialists utilize this image as the Reiki treatment is finishing, settling the body and fixing the stirred qi inside. The striking lightning jolt image made by the hands attracts a descending motion, symbolizing the finishing of the recuperating session.

## THE POWER SYMBOLS

The Mental/Emotional image – Sei He Ki
 (Sei He Ki articulated as: "State Hay-Key")
Sei He Ki has a general importance of: "God and man become one".

The Mental/Emotional image unites the "cerebrum and the body". It encourages individuals to bring to the surface and discharge the psychological/enthusiastic reasons for their issues.

Numerous individuals (even specialists) are beginning to understand that many of our diseases depend on mental and enthusiastic unbalances that we presumably are not by any means mindful of. The image attempts to center and blend the subliminal with the physical side.

This image can be utilized to help with enthusiastic and mental mending. It adjusts the left and right half of the cerebrum and gives harmony and amicability. It is additionally exceptionally successful on relationship issues. The Sei He Ki image can likewise be utilized on different issues like apprehension, dread, gloom, outrage, pity and so forth.


**A few clearings:**

The images can be utilized to help mend abuse of medications, liquor, smoking and so on.

Sei He Ki can be utilized to get in shape.


The image can be utilized to discover things that you have lost. (Attract the image front of you and request help in discovering it. Relinquish attempting to discover the item. The appropriate response will before long spring up). Sei He Ki can be utilized to improve your memory when perusing and contemplating. Draw the image on each page as you read it with the goal of recollecting the significant parts. Include the image when doing healing (normal or distance) as this can support the mending procedure. Numerous physical issues have mental/enthusiastic roots.

## Additional data

The Mental/Emotional image, Sei He Ki, has to do with Yin and Yang and the harmony between the different sides of the cerebrum.

The left piece of the image speaks to Yang and our left half of the cerebrum (rational, structure and straight reasoning and so forth). The right side of the image speaks to Yin and our right side of the mind (dreams, sentiments, instincts and so on). When you are confronting someone else and draw the image the left half of the image, for example the Yang part of the image winds up on the collector's correct side of the cerebrum and the Yin part on the left side in this way adjusting the different sides.

Reiki symbols are fundamentally words from Japanese language that assume a significant job in Reiki practice. These images are utilized by cutting edge Reiki specialists and can help in centering or directing the Reiki energies. The images can be initiated either by imagining them rationally, drawing the image with the palm of your hand, talking the name of the image for all to hear or basically conjuring it in your brain. The three essential images utilized in conventional Reiki are Cho Ku Rei (control symbol), Sei He Ki (mental or passionate mending symbol) and Hon Sha Ze Sho Nen (separation recuperating image).

### What meaning does Sei He Ki have?

"Sei He Ki" means "The Earth and Sky meet or God and Man become one". This image follows up on an individual's cognizant personality (the psychological body) and subliminal personality (passionate body) and is utilized fundamentally for enthusiastic and mental mending, clearing, purging, assurance and adjusting. Occasionally it's called "The Protection Symbol", in view of the role it plays in giving assurance. A large portion of our illnesses are caused by mental and psychical irregularity in our bodies. The utilization of the enthusiastic mending image helps in carrying the issue to the surface and frees mental issues. This image likewise helps in adjusting the left and right half of the mind and advances harmony and agreement. It tends to be utilized to draw delicate and unobtrusive energies required to facilitate the sentiments of distress or resistence.

### The most effective method to Use the Reiki Emotional/Mental Symbol

Various specialists utilize this image in various ways. For instance, the specialist draws the Cho Ku Rei (the control image) to make an association with the Reiki vitality source. Sei He Ki is however drawn over the pained territory where the Reiki energies are required. The energies are fixed by drawing the power image or Cho Ku Rei once more. This supports the impact of Sei He Ki for a more extended time.

### Improving Memory Power

Sei He Ki is valuable in improving your memory. Drawing this Reiki image on pages of your book, can enable you to retain the substance while studying or examining. Envisioning the image over your head can enable you to recollect things that you may have overlooked, for example your keys, the name of an individual, an answer for the test, or pretty much whatever else. This works as a result of the associations this image makes in between the two halves of the brain.

### Saying No to Bad Habits

The psychological image helps in reestablishing passionate and mental equalization in an individual's body and advances profound healing. The utilization of this Reiki image helps in taking out undesirable or unfortunate propensities such liquor addiction, smoking cigarettes or gorging. Imagining or drawing this Reiki image around you helps in changing your pessimistic convictions, adverse parental or social molding and makes you an increasingly constructive individual.

### Improving Relationships

Drawing Sei He Ki around your environment and the individuals associated with a grieved relationship can achieve the intelligence and solidarity to graciously deal with issues. Utilizing this Reiki image will help carry relationship issues to the surface and make you handle them effectively.

### Enabling Your Affirmations

Certifications are useful assets that can assume a crucial job in helping you to accomplish your objective effectively. The psychological image works in the intuitive personality. Rehashing the name of this image rationally can help in strengthening your perseverance and achieving your objective.

### Individual Bodyguard

Drawing Sei He Ki around you helps shielding you from the negative vibrations and enabling just the positive energies to contact you. As referenced, it is generally called the protection image and can likewise be utilized as a defensive shield during cleansing functions to help in expelling negative energy from the physical body.

In therapeutic settings, this image will in general fill in as a "sterile balm", when utilized previously, during or after an activity or medical procedure.

## Dispersing Headaches

Sei He Ki is utilized to heal intense subject matters that can cause physical issues as well. By utilizing this Reiki image, you can figure out how to mend your cerebral pain caused due to any psychological precariousness. This may very well be a way to fix your migraines normally, without taking any sort of drugs (make sure to drink a big quantity of water as well, since many types of cerebral pain are caused by lack of hydration).

## Discovering Lost Objects

Drawing the Reiki mental image in front of you and requesting help to find lost articles will help you either discover the items or give you capacity to think and recall the area where you kept them.

## Harmony

This image shows us the synchronization or harmony of things in nature. It teaches us about the musical cycle of nature, the need of versatility towards changes and understanding the significance of non-connection. It shows a more inspirational viewpoint of life and helps individuals to remain grateful for longer time.

# CHAPTER 6
# THE HEALING OF REIKI

Numerous individuals are rehearsing strategies to improve their wellbeing, for example, reflection, exercise and improved eating routine. As this is done, a more profound mindfulness frequently creates, concerning the progression of inconspicuous energies in and around the body and the association between these unobtrusive energies and one's wellbeing. This mindfulness approves the antiquated thought of 'life power vitality' as the reason for wellbeing and its need as the reason for disease. The presence of 'life power vitality' and the need for it to stream openly in and around one's body to keep up wellbeing has been contemplated and recognized by medicinal services specialists just as researchers.

Our body is made not just out of physical components, as muscles, bones, nerves, veins, organs, and so on. It likewise has an inconspicuous vitality framework through which 'life power vitality' streams. This unpretentious vitality framework is made of energy 'bodies' that enclose our physical body and help us in handling our contemplations and feelings. The energy bodies have vitality focuses called chakras, which work fairly like valves that allow life power to circle through the physical, mental, passionate and profound bodies. We have vitality meridians and nadas. These resemble waterways or streams, which convey our life power vitality all through our physical body, to feed us and help with adjusting our body's strcture and capacities.

Our physical body is alive and active due to the 'existence power vitality' that is streaming. Assuming our 'life power' is low or blocked, we are bound to become ill, however if it is high and free streaming, we all the more effectively keep up wellbeing and a sentiment of prosperity. One thing that upsets and debilitates the progression of 'life power vitality' is pressure. Stress is frequently brought up by clashing introspections and emotions that get held up in one's unobtrusive vitality framework. These incorporate panic, stress, questions, outrage, tension and so on. Medicinal research has verified that nonstop pressure can hinder the body's normal capacity to fix, recover and ensure itself. The American Institute of Stress appraises that 75%-95% of all visits to specialists are the consequences of response to attacks. The impacts of unreleased pressure extend from minor longs to significant wellbeing concerns, for example, coronary illnesses, stomach related issues, respiratory and skin issues.

Reiki (beam key) is a strategy that guides the body in discharging pressure and tension through profound unwinding. Along these lines, Reiki advances healing and wellbeing. The word "Reiki" comes from two Japanese words – "Rei" which signifies "the Wisdom of God or the Higher Power" and "Ki" which means "life power vitality". So, Reiki signifies 'profoundly guided life power vitality.' The Reiki plan of healing is a method for transmitting this inconspicuous vitality to yourself as well as other people through the hands into the human vitality structure. Reiki reestablishes vitality unity and imperativeness by appeasing the physical and passionate impacts of unreleased pressure. It delicately and adequately opens blocked meridians, nadas and chakras and clears the energy bodies, leaving one's capability loose and settled.

**What Reiki can do for you:**

- it accelerates healing.
- It gives assistance to the body by cleansing toxins.
- It balances the flow of subtle energy by releasing blockages.
- Reiki helps the client contact the 'healer within.'

A treatment feels like warm, delicate daylight that moves through you, surrounds you and comforts you. Reiki treats the individual's body, feelings, psyche and soul in general. Reiki is a straightforward, normal and safe technique for profound recovery and personal development that everybody can utilize.

Reiki is amazing, yet magnificently delicate and supporting. During a treatment, the customers remain completely dressed. Reiki is a successful option or supplement to the Knead treatment. Reiki supports any medicinal or supplemental mending technique a customer might utilize and encourages chiropractors, restorative specialists, physiotherapists, psychotherapists, therapists and trance inducers.

Anybody can figure out how to take advantage of a boundless stock of 'life power vitality' to improve wellbeing and upgrade the personal satisfaction by learning Reiki or by accepting medication from a Reiki Practitioner or Master.

Reiki, the mending treatment invented by a Japanese Buddhist named Mikao Usui over a hundred years ago, depends on a basic profound standard: We're altogether guided by the equivalent undetectable life power and it controls our physical, mental and passionate prosperity. When the energy streams openly, we can take advantage of mysterious reserves of intensity. When it keeps running into blockages (frequently said to be brought up by negative reasoning, unhealed injuries, or stress over-burden), we work at an imperfect level.

While this may seem like voodoo enchantment to a few, even nonbelievers who have gone through an hour with a talented Reiki ace (as they're called) have felt a positive move or some likeness thereof. Many depict Reiki sessions—a mix of light touch or energy clearing—as quieting or establishing. Furthermore, for other people, it feels like a passionate realignment.

Reiki aces, as Kelsey Patel, train for quite a long time to comprehend and explore vitality shifts, however Patel says anybody can adapt (rapidly) to work with vitality and enforce the progression of others.

## Initial Step: Receiving Energy

To start any Reiki practice, you should actuate the vitality inside yourself. Close your eyes and take some rounds of full breaths. Envision the crown of your head opening and a surge of mending white light spilling out of the highest point of your head, into your heart and out through your arms and hands. Request to be filled where you need mending most. Along these lines, in case you're going to offer Reiki to a friend or family member, you won't serve them from an empty cup.

As you feel the progression of vitality, proceed to inhale and assuming you discover your psyche gets occupied or begins to address whether this is working, breathe out. Imagine yourself as a boat of healing.

## Reiki for Sleep

To give a rest centered Reiki session to a companion or relative, have them rest while you position yourself close to their head. Envision a constant flow of recuperating light going from your hands into the back of their head and clearing the psyche of any agony or distress encountered that day.

Request that your cherished one takes a few rounds of full breaths and gradually alternates an inhalation of three seconds and an exhalation of three to five seconds.

Ask them to gradually observe an image at once and to thank every memory before releasing it with their breath.

Enable them to float off as you keep on directing the vitality through your palms and send the healing light into their whole body. Envision the body getting to be mended, loose and comfortable for a calm night rest. You can offer this Reiki for as long as you need, yet fifteen to thirty minutes should be enough for them to feel loose and serene.

## Reiki for Stress

Frequently when individuals have uneasiness and stress, they are not breathing appropriately and the brevity of breath can cause more pressure. In this Reiki session, you need to channel vitality down the beneficiary's shoulders and into their body. Place your hands on their shoulders for ten to fifteen minutes. Concentrate on sending vitality into their entire body and breathing profoundly with them. This can normally bring a portion of the serious mental energy down and get it once more into their body. Assuming your patient is resting, you can put your hands behind their head, as well, to enable them to quiet down.

I suggest staying in a similar spot for fifteen to twenty minutes for extreme unwinding.

## Last Step: Sealing Off Energy

It's essential to offer appreciation, purge yourself and close the vitality once you've finished a mending session. It very well may be as straightforward as venturing back, cleaning your hands of any overabundance of vitality and setting them in prayer position to express gratitude towards yourself, the vitality and the beneficiary for the trade. You can likewise draw an enormous circle, crossing the arms before the body to mean the end of your two energies and closure with hands in imploration.

## A Note on Adults versus Kids

In case you're offering Reiki to your partner or different grown-ups, recollect that a few adults, after some time, have overlooked how to feel (or have turned out to be less mindful of) their vivacious and physical body. That is alright. Simply realize that they may state they can't feel the vitality moving. It may be inconspicuous, yet it doesn't imply that your vitality didn't influence them.

When working with children, depending upon their age, you can likewise share with them what you are doing and why. Children are exceptionally discerning and will, in general, be unfathomably open to elective practices. A few guardians will likewise tell youngsters the best way to get vitality and do Reiki themselves, so they start to get to their gateway to recuperating at an early age.

## SIGNIFICANCE OF REIKI AS AN ALTERNATIVE MEDICINE

Reiki is a kind of vitality mending that was created in Japan by Dr Mikao Usui. A Reiki expert will utilize light touch which expects to change and adjust the vitality fields in and around your body.

### Outline

· The Japanese word Reiki implies all-inclusive vitality.

· It plans to loosen you up, ease pressure and strain and help your general prosperity.

· A Reiki expert will utilize recuperating vitality by laying their hands on your dressed body.

· You may also hear it's named Reiki vitality, Usui arrangement of Reiki and helpful touch.

The Japanese word Reiki implies all-inclusive vitality. Eastern drug structures work with this vitality, which courses through every single living thing and is indispensable to prosperity. The vitality is known as 'Ki' in Japan, 'Chi' in China and 'prana' in India. Reiki isn't a piece of a religion or conviction. It is best portrayed as a type of hands on healing utilized as a reciprocal treatment.

A Reiki specialist intends to change and adjust the vitality fields in and around your body to help on a physical, mental, enthusiastic and otherworldly level.

**Reiki professionals state that it can:**

· help you feel profoundly loose;

· help you adapt to troublesome circumstances;

· soothe enthusiastic pressure and strain;

· ensure improvements in general prosperity.

A few people with diseases state they feel better in the wake of utilizing treatments, for example, Reiki. Studies demonstrate this is regularly in light of the fact that an advisor invests energy with the individual and contacts them.

After the anxiety and fear of being in emergency clinics and under treatment, it very well may be extremely loosening up when somebody gives you consideration for an hour or more, in a quiet setting. Reiki is sometimes utilized in palliative application, particularly in hospices.

A few people say that Reiki has controlled symptoms of their medication, for example torment, uneasiness and affliction.

They likewise state that it causes them to adapt better to their disease and its treatment. In any case, it's essential to understand that while Reiki may assist you with coping with your treatments or symptoms, it can't treat your desease.

**How you have it**

On your first visit, your Reiki professional will get some information about your general wellbeing and medical history. They might ask you for why you want to have Reiki and talk about your treatment plan with you.

You don't need to get undressed for treatment. You may often need to take your shoes and coat off. You can have your eyes open or shut.

Your Reiki specialist may lower the lights or play relieving music. They will put their hands on, or a couple of inches over your body. They will move their hands over your body, typically beginning at your head and working down to your feet, yet may concentrate on specific areas of the body.

The point is to move and adjust the vitality inside and around your body. Furthermore, to arrange any energy source in order to reinforce your vitality.

You may feel a shivering sensation, a profound unwinding, warmth or coolness all through your body. Or then again, you probably won't feel anything by any stretch of the imagination. Specialists state this doesn't mean the treatment isn't working.

So, a session for the most part keeps going between 20 minutes and 60 minutes. Numerous professionals state you will get the best outcomes from 3 sessions on a short period of time. At that point enjoy a reprieve before having more medicines.

You may feel thirsty after a session. You need to drink a lot of water and stay away from solid caffeine-based beverages, for example espresso.

You may feel profoundly loose and resting at home for a while can enable you to get the full advantage of the treatment.

Reiki can be performed at a distance. A fittingly prepared specialist can send mending afar. So, you can be in your own home having Reiki from an individual somewhere else.

## Symptoms

As a rule, Reiki is alright for many people suffering from different diseases. Most experts will encourage you to rest and drink a lot of water after the treatment. There are no reports of unsafe symptoms.

It is safe to have Reiki when under treatment for tumors. However, it's essential to inform your PCP regarding any correlative treatment, elective treatment or diet supplement that you use. However, at that point your primary care physician will consistently have the full picture about your consideration and treatment.

Reiki (霊気) is a kind of elective prescription called vitality healing. Reiki experts use a technique called palm recuperating or hands-on mending through which "widespread vitality" is said to be moved through the palms of the master to the patient to engage mental or physical healing.

## Significance:

Reiki leads different analysis: the physical, mental, spiritual and otherworldly, restoring everything. One of the best Reiki circumstances are pressure drop and unwinding, which triggers the body's characteristic recuperating limits (safe framework), helps rest and wellbeing.

## 1. Effectively supports Harmony and Balance

Reiki accelerates harmony and consistency. It is a viable, non-obtrusive vitality mending technique that updates the body's common recuperating limit while empowering and propelling wellbeing. Reiki works explicitly on reestablishing peace on all levels and works directly on the issue and condition as opposed to just concealing.

When we talk about equalization, we mean mental and spiritual parity, left and right personality, masculine and feminine, naming things as incredible or awful, constructive or adverse etc.

## 2. Brings profound relaxation and empowers the body to discharge melancholy and anxiety

What numerous individuals acknowledge about Reiki treatment is it grants them uninterrupted alone time where they aren't 'doing' yet essentially 'being'. Clients have displayed predilection for being clearer, more calm, loose and lighter.

Reiki gives a space where you can be increasingly mindful of what's going on inside your body and brain, to figure out how to tune in to your very own body and choose savvy decisions, concerning your thriving from this spot. Being increasingly present implies you are in your body, which urges you to get to significantly more than internal information and knowledge that you have.

## 3. Separates energy areas and advances characteristic harmony between mind, body and soul

Standard Reiki treatment can mean a progressively settled and increasingly peaceful state of being, in which an individual is better prepared to adapt to ordinary pressure. This mental equalization likewise improves learning, memory and mental clearness.

Reiki can mend mental/spiritual wounds and can help ease emotional episodes, fear, disappointment and even outrage. Reiki can likewise fortify and heal individual bonds.

Since Reiki improves your ability to cherish, it can open you up to the individuals around you and help you bound with them.

## 4. Helps the body in purifying itself from toxic substances and supports the resistant framework

We put so much energy in stress-responsive reactions that it transforms into our 'standard' and our bodies really disregard how to return to change.

Reiki reminds our bodies how to move into a parasympathetic tactile framework (rest/process) self-patching mode.

## 5. Helps significant advancement and excited cleansing

You don't have to be into spirituality to welcome the benefits of Reiki. Nonetheless, for a few, they get Reiki cures to help themselves through their self-mending adventure, for instance significant advancement/personal development.

Reiki addresses the whole being, instead of concentrating on individual signs.

It can emphasize simple developments inside your very own being. What does that look like? Concentrating on irritating conditions can come even more effectively.

Reiki is a successful technique for self-healing and vitality restoration and, more so, can be a great weight-loss technique.

Reiki is an elective wellbeing treatment that permits mending through the channeling and move of widespread crucial vitality that streams all through the body, subsequently wiping out conceivable mental and emotional imbalances.

The utilization of Reiki as a technique to get thinner has incredible advantages since overweight isn't just activated by poor eating habits, yet in addition by an inactive way of life and spiritual issues, for example uneasiness, stress, sorrow, disappointment, among others. What's more, this is unequivocally what Reiki can heal.

The progression of general indispensable vitality through our body enables us to adjust inside and from that point divert our will, quieting those habitual practices that lead us to an unfortunate eating routine.

**Reiki activities to get in shape:**

First position: Just place your hands on the sides of your head, as though holding it tenderly, close your eyes, and inhale profoundly in harmony.

Second position: inhale and breathe out a few times and envision how you might want to see yourself. Along these lines, you will attract into your life every one of the progressions and objectives you need to accomplish.

Third position: place the hands close to the throat, without contacting it, to control the emission of thyroid hormones and increment the basal metabolic rate.

Fourth position: place two hands in the navel area, with the fingers crossed. Along these lines the vitality streams more effectively and permits to cleanse and detoxify the hurtful substances.

Fifth position: just put your hands on your knees and inhale profoundly. This will help accelerate blood flow in the legs, improve lymphatic drainage and advance liquid preservation.

Keep going position: put your hands on one of your feet, one on the base and another on the instep. In this position you will wash down the life condition. You should repeat this system with the other foot.

## SELF HEALING

A Reiki expert fundamentally replaces an individual's life power with their own, from one part of the body into the other person's root chakra. Reiki works based on the idea that people are vitality vessels and that this vitality is transmutable.

## GATHERING HEALING AND HEALING OTHERS WITH REIKI

You can begin mending other individuals directly in the wake of being sensitive to Reiki. As a Reiki 1 level, you should be close to the patient you are helping. After Reiki 2, besides hands-on healing, you can send anybody Reiki, regardless of their location.

### Hands-On Healing

When you are giving hands-on healing to somebody, you can either have them sit or rest. Making them rest is the most advantageous, both for the healer and the patient, as the healer gets access to all chakras and the patient can unwind totally.

If you speak to the patient before, request that they wear baggy garments. At the moment of the procedure, request that they take off their watch, jewelry, belt and so on. Gold and silver jewels might be worn. Ensure you and the patient both drink a glass of water.

Request that they calmly rest on their back and close their eyes. Start by mending the crown/forehead chakra and afterward keep on healing all the front chakras.

When done, balance the energy by spiraling. This means to keep your left hand on their right shoulder and with your right hand (index and center finger expanded, thumb contacting the ring and little finger) draw counterclockwise spirals beginning from the left shoulder, to the tip of the left hand. Next, draw the spirals from the left shoulder to the left foot, at that point from the right shoulder to the right foot and afterwards, right shoulder to the tip of the right hand.

Have the patient turn over the right side and lie on their stomach. Concentrate on the back chakras.

The following stage is balancing. Hold your hands over the back temples and back root chakras, around 6 inches over the body. Attempt to feel the irregularity of energies and give Reiki till the vitality levels feel balanced. At that point move your hands gradually to the back throat and back hara chakras. Once these chakras are likewise adjusted, move gradually to the back heart and back sun powered chakras. At the point when these two chakras are adjusted, bring both your hands over the heart chakra and rest it over the body.

Keep your left hand on the patient's left shoulder. With the index and center finger of your right hand, create a V shape and draw a line from the throat to the root chakra. At that point draw a line from the root to the throat chakra. Rest your right hand on his/her back hara chakra. Do this three times. Tenderly shake the patient.

**Distance Healing**

Distance mending should be possible by channels who are sensitive to Reiki 2 or above. When you are giving afar healing to somebody, it is smarter to request that they set some time apart to get the energy you send them. This expands their vitality assimilation and will to heal themselves. Demand that they sit with their eyes shut, uncovered feet contacting the floor, without touching their hands or legs. Give them a chance to attempt to feel the vitality coming to them.

There are a few different ways of sending energy from a distance. You could utilize an item as a photo, a tag, envision them or send them Reiki through your third eye. Every one of these focal points needs to be analyzed in detail.

# Far away Healing Techniques

### Utilizing a Photograph

You could ask the patient for a photo and send Reiki vitality to the equivalent. Draw the images on the back of the photo and if there is enough space, you may even write above it that their concern is understood. Hold the photo between your palms and envision the images on it while giving Reiki.

### Utilizing a Surrogate

You could utilize a stuffed toy or a comparable item as a surrogate. Rationally affirm the toy to be the patient and start giving it Reiki. You can offer Reiki to the targeted part or give full body Reiki to it. You could likewise proclaim little items or your thumb as the patient and hold it between your palms and give Reiki.

## Creative mind

Keep your palms together and envision the individual either inside your palms or in front of you, accepting the vitality you send and washing in it. Envision them feeling better and draw the images while giving them Reiki.

## Third Eye

Assuming the individual is noticeable, you can envision Reiki vitality getting through your third eye and setting off to that individual. Envision a light emission turning out through your third eye and draw the images on them with that bar. You could utilize this system when you are taking a glimpse at their photo or basically envisioning that they are standing in front of you and accepting Reiki through your third eye.

## Promise Slip

You could have a promise box, something that can fit into your palm and contain papers. Take a little piece of paper and compose your prediction on one side. Make sure to utilize just positive words (abstain from utilizing 'no', 'not', 'don't', 'won't', 'can't', and so forth), keep away from any full stops (period ) and don't crease the paper. After the conclusion, end it with 'It is in this way, Thank you Reiki, Thy will be finished'. On the other side of the paper, draw every one of the images. Move it up and put it in the goal box.

The positive aspect of the goal box is that you can offer Reiki to many individuals/occasions simultaneously. At whatever point you wish, hold the container between your palms, rationally draw the images on it and give Reiki. You don't need to think about every one of the expectations independently.

## Far off Healing for Events

You can send far off healing for occasions and events. Far off recuperating can likewise be sent for mending and fixing broken connections.

Intension papers and creative mind methods can be utilized for this sort of mending. You can likewise rationally repeat: 'X occasion is fruitful. It is thus, Thank You Reiki, Thy will be done' while giving Reiki. The main line might be substituted with various proclamations relying upon the condition.

Reiki can likewise be used for past occasions which still hurt/have any kind of repercussion in your life. This is particularly useful for those with youth injuries and broken connections. Reiki can't change the past, yet it will change the way you feel about the occasion being referred to and furthermore encourage you to forgive the individuals in question.

## Reiki by Consent

A typical uncertainty of Reiki channels is whether you can offer Reiki to others without their consent. This situation can be understood, assuming you have a reasonable picture regarding WHY consent is required in any case.

When an individual gives you his accord for Reiki, two significant things are occurring subliminally. Right off the bat, by consenting, he is opening himself up to any vitality that you may send his way. Besides, and even more critically, consenting additionally advises his subliminal personality to begin getting ready to be healed and his very own body begins effectively attempting to mend itself.

Even though it is difficult to acknowledge, we are never wiped out except if we genuinely need to be. We are talking at an inner mind level here, because intentionally, we frequently appear to be totally tired of our sickness. In such cases, assent sets the way for a quicker recuperation. When somebody requests Reiki, they are requesting help to improve and that itself sends a major message to their subconscious.

In situations when you don't request an individual's assent, that individual keeps on staying in the equivalent mental and intuitive condition of happiness and it is a lot harder and takes longer, if at all he is restored. Hence, we energize taking assent.

If an individual is in a condition of obviousness or in some other manner unable to consent, it is right to send cherishing Reiki vitality their way. In situations where you need to free someone else of fixation or sickness without/against their assent, improvement might be irrelevant.

## Free Reiki

Regardless of whether Reiki needs to be given for free or not is profoundly discussed among Reiki specialists. As indicated by the legend, Mikao Usui stated that Reiki shall not be offered for free, after his unpleasant involvement with the poor people in the ghettos of Kyoto. He felt that anything given free of expense isn't esteemed. Some sort of vitality trade needs to exist, either in real money, kindness or administration, as a byproduct of Reiki mending. Consequently, you can generally offer Reiki to family and dear companions, since they effectively take an interest in energy exchanges with you once a day.

In any case, others accept that we get vitality and help from different individuals, sometimes outsiders, who don't charge us and we should freely give Reiki as nature will adjust the vitality. They accept that it doesn't make a difference whether an individual quantifies Reiki or the treatment and that they should progress in the direction of helping other people without requesting something in exchange.

The vast majority view Reiki as holy and not to be given away for free. They argue that one doesn't give away gold for nothing, at that point why Reiki? Reiki given for free is viewed as philanthropy, much along the lines of free sustenance or garments. They often charge a fixed expense and if the patient is excessively poor, charge a day's pay or some work in exchange.

Both these perspectives are not off base, as each Reiki channel is guided by Reiki. If you are in difficulty, let Reiki be your guide and pursue your instinct.

Even though it is preferable, a complete Reiki session conditions can emerge that will avert Reiki specialists from having the option to give somebody a full treatment. In any occasion, a shorter session is better than none by any means.

Here are the fundamental hand positions for experts to use in doing an abbreviated Reiki session. As opposed to setting down on a bed, love seat or back rub table the patient sits upstanding in a seat. Similar directions apply, assuming you are expecting to offer Reiki to somebody blocked in a wheelchair.

## Essential Instructions for Carrying Out a Quick Session

Have the customer sit in a straight upheld seat or wheelchair. Instruct your customer to take a few deep loosening up breaths. Take a couple of profound purifying breaths yourself too. Continue with your treatment starting with the shoulder position. These hands positions are expected to be utilized with your palms touching the patient's body. Nonetheless, you can likewise apply non-contact Reiki treatment by floating your hands two or three inches from the body by following these equivalent motions.

**Shoulder Position -** Standing behind the customer, place each one of your hands over their shoulders. (2-5 minutes)

**Top of Head Position** - Lay your palms on the highest point of the head, hands level, thumbs contacting. (2-5 minutes)

**Medulla Oblongata/Forehead Position** - Move to the customer's side, lay one hand on the Medulla oblongata (the region between the back of the head and the highest point of the spine) and the other on the temple. (2-5 minutes)

**Vertebra/Throat Position** - Lay one hand on the seventh projecting cervical vertebra and the other in the pit of the throat. (2-5 minutes)

**Back/Breastbone Position** - Lay one hand on the breastbone and the other on the back at the equivalent height. (2-5 minutes)

**Back/Solar Plexus Position** - Lay one hand on the sun-oriented plexus (stomach) and the other at a similar tallness on the back. (2-5 minutes)

**Back/Lower Stomach Position** - Lay one hand on the lower stomach and the other at the base of the back at a similar tallness. (2-5 minutes)

**Auric Sweep** - Finish with an emanation clearing to purify the auric field of the patient's body. (1 moment)

**Supportive Tips:**

If the patient needs the support of the back of the seat through the session, basically lay your hand on the back of the seat as opposed to laying it onto the body. Reiki energy will naturally penetrate through the seat to the individual. This is particularly great to know, if you are working with a customer who is in a wheelchair.

Be sure that you have enough time to perform a full treatment, do your best not to give the feeling that you are hurrying. Utilize the brief span accessible to you in a quiet condition of unwinding.

Reiki hand positions are unspoken rules, but don't hesitate to change the grouping or adjust the positions naturally or in the manner that feels fitting.

Ensure you (the facilitator) are enjoying the session too, regardless of whether you are seated or standing. It can get very tedious to do a seat treatment from a standing position - twisting around, and so on.

Book a follow-up treatment for your patient.

## Reiki First Aid

Reiki was also proven to be amazing as an extra method for giving first aid in case of misfortunes. Here you should quickly lay one hand onto the sun-based plexus and the other onto the kidneys (suprarenal organs). When you have done this, move the second hand to the external edge of the shoulders.

# CHAPTER 7
# THE POWER OF REIKI TO ATTRACT ANYTHING YOU WANT

**Attracting Your Soul Mate with Reiki**

Smetimes your most noteworthy soul-level development originates from being single and some of the time it originates from being in a relationship. There is somebody who is an ideal vibrational pair for you. Simply have tolerance and trust the celestial planning.

## GETTING OUT THE OLD ENERGY

Reiki won't just enable you to attract a perfect partner, it will enable you to clear your relationship patterns that don't serve you. You can utilize Reiki to get out your vitality in the wake of cutting off an association.

By utilizing Reiki on yourself to end up mindful and discharge your wrong patterns, you will make place for a really new relationship. The main consistent factor in the entirety of your connections is "You". With Reiki, you can calibrate yourself to be the most ideal You, to draw in the perfect accomplice for you.

For instance, say you simply cut off a relationship with somebody who you were satisfied with. If you don't clear your vibration of factious vitality, you'll end up in another antagonistic partnership. Obviously, you may not see this until after the newness wears off. In case you're yet a vibrational match to belligerence, that is the thing that you'll appeal to.

With Reiki you can clear the energy in you that vibrates with conflict, so you're never again a vibrational match to it (or whatever undesired relationship feature you've been experiencing). That way, when you start another relationship it will be like a breath of fresh air. You can make a holy space with your new darling to reflect your present and new degree of vibration.

Here's only one thought for an approach to get out an old enthusiastic example:

Reiki yourself while envisioning the Reiki vacuuming ceaselessly all the energy of your past relationship that doesn't serve you anymore. It very well may be a sure characteristic like struggle, exploiting someone or sentiments of abandonment. Use Reiki to release any undesirable energy while staying open for individual bits of knowledge and mindfulness into your relationship patterns.

When you sense that you have gotten out all the undesired force, empower yourself to be loaded up with Reiki and qualities that help you find yourself, like coherence strength and feeling connected with your awesome self.

## ACKNOWLEDGING BEING SINGLE

Reiki will likewise help you in genuinely valuing the time between relationships. Reiki can enlighten your spirit level desires and interests carrying them to the cutting edge, so you'll recollect what's imperative to your spirit level way throughout everyday life. With Reiki, you'll get clear on viewpoints you are not willing to settle on in your next relationship.

Reiki can enable you to figure out how to enjoy being in connection with yourself as you treat yourself as you would a dearest one. What an incredible method to sustain yourself by utilizing the cherishing and supporting vitality of Reiki. The more profound your self-esteem, the more profound your ability to cherish another.

## DEVELOPING PATIENCE AND TRUST

You've done your internal work and are emanating your adoring self. Presently you are prepared to pull in your adoring perfect partner. Maybe you've just begun sending Reiki to be meeting him/her. You're going to social events that you're drown to. Still no karma.

Make sure to send Reiki to yourself and develop persistence and trust in perfect planning. When you are an ideal vibrational match to meeting somebody, you will.

## ASSOCIATING ON THE SPIRITUAL LEVEL

You can utilize Reiki to associate with your perfect partner on the profound level before you meet in the physical one. Once you are sensitive to the subsequent degree, utilize the far-off image to interfere with the energy of your next perfect sweetheart, regardless of whether it be your perfect partner or twin soul. Expect connecting to them in the astral plane during your fantasies.

In case you're a Reiki 1, just Reiki yourself with the goal to be profoundly connected with your optimal, cherishing mate during your rest.

Simply appreciate the sentiment of interacting while, at the same time, relishing sentiments of soul-level love. Maybe you'll recollect previous existence connections or looks at soul level recollections.

Try not to get up to speed attempting to make sense of where, when and how you meet in the physical. Getting concentrated on points of interest will probably put you in a condition of obstruction. If you get a few incredible subtleties, the primary concern of interacting with your crush on the otherworldly horizon remains to feel the affection and establish a feeling of confidence and trust.

## GETTING TO HOOK UP WITH YOUR SOUL MATE

Continue sending Reiki without connection to when, where and how. Remain open to the direction you're given. There's no set-in stone manner to meet. In case you're propelled to online dating, put it all on the line. Assuming you simply realize that you're intended to go to an event, at that point purchase your ticket.

Keep your consideration on adoring yourself and emanating who you genuinely are. There's nothing more alluring than somebody sparkling their spirit level self.

Trust that you'll know in your heart and mind that you've met your cherishing half. You may feel this knowing from the start or maybe after numerous years. Realize that you are love and have the right to be cherished.

## It's All About Self-Healing

Figuring out how to pull in positive things into your life is about self-healing on the spiritual and otherworldly levels.

Here's a straightforward "math". When you don't experience plenitude of affection or cash, then it implies the progression of reward into your life is blocked. Why is it so? What squares are? All things considered, they are negative feelings, terrible recollections, negative convictions about cash or love, dread, stress, concerns, anarchic personality, diversions – every one of these things hinder the progression of wealth. Assuming you wish to encounter abundance in your life, you need to self-mend the things that fit you. This is possible through Reiki. At the point when every one of the squares is gone, you start to find your own gifts, characteristic capacities and aptitudes – every one of the things that later on can be re-made into monetary steadiness, for instance by propelling your own business.

What's more, with the squares like stresses or fears gone, you start to acknowledge life. More positive feelings stream into your life, considering this fact, the excellence was consistently there around you – just now without the squares in your psyche, you're ready to see it. Through recuperating, you see magnificence and openings and the plenitude that is now around you.

Along these lines, for instance if there should be an occurrence of pulling in budgetary wellbeing: first, you must mend all your negative convictions about money. Then, you build up your internal gifts and capacities, that will enable you to profit, build up self-esteem, which will attract adoration, companions and, lastly, bliss. Basic :).

Some of such negative convictions or examples or obstructions that keep you down, were clarified in a book - "Wealth through Reiki"

What's more, mending is done through the standard routine with regards to ordinary and straightforward Reiki.

## There is no Magical Reiki Symbol

In all actuality there is no otherworldly Reiki image for cash, nor is there a Reiki image for affection and so forth. Indeed, we may discover such images related to Reiki, however in most cases, they are portions of nowadays Reiki systems such as Gold Reiki, Kundalini Reiki and others. In the conventional method for Reiki we have just four images – CKR, SHK, HSZSN and DKM. None of these is intended explicitly to pull in cash into our financial balance.

There is straightforward, no mystical and quick approach to utilize Reiki to draw in cash or love. There is just a more extended way – the way of self-healing. But in the event of otherworldly mending, the quick ways never work over the long run and the genuine healing requires some serious energy. Once you have realized there is no mystical path around here, you can start to acknowledge that, assuming you wish to attract cash or love through Reiki, you have to put in two or three months, sometimes even years, on working with Reiki to mend yourself. And, when you're prepared to acknowledge this, Reiki will really enable you to achieve your goals.

**Approaches to Use Reiki to Attract Abundance**

If wish to utilize Reiki to attract wealth, at that point you can pursue these tips and practices day by day. With time – and indeed, that implies weeks, months, lastly years – you will see that your life improves.

Work with mending affirmations – either with Reiki or without Reiki, the healing attestations will work. I've distributed two or three articles both here on *Reiki Paths* and on *A State of Mind*.

Look for books on plenitude, abundance and love – many writers shared books that talk about the manners in which we see wealth, cash or love. Part of these books are healing books, pointing to us our negative convictions that must be mended, giving us tips on mending and dproving to us the positive things we should begin to accept.

Perform self-Reiki often – with the goal of healing everything that keeps you from encountering love or abundance. Also, be persistent, because once you set the goal and simply let Reiki stream, this otherworldly power will continue healing you.

Work with Five Reiki Precepts –at whatever point you experience negative thoughs or feelings about cash or love or anything you wish to bring into your life, consider these things from the viewpoint of the Precepts. Consideration can discharge more contemplations, recollections or feelings that square the progression of plenitude into your life.

Work with the initial two symbols –the CKR and the SHK. The main image is an establishing image. Its job is to ground us and give us the feeling of material safety, which additionally manages material apprehensions. The subsequent image causes us to mend our feelings and negative mental propensities, that additionally incorporate negative convictions or practices that inhibit the progression of affection or wealth. It likewise causes us to "open up our heart" which is significant for the individuals who wish to attract love.

Make a Reiki Box – make a case. At that point write your desires or dreams on little bits of paper and place them in the case. "Give it Reiki" every day, send Reiki into the box with the goal of accomplishing the fantasies and objectives and things you've written on the papers. Each time you do so, review these composed objectives and be grateful that Reiki helps you accomplish them.

Practice Reiki manifestation – a instructional exercise has been shared on *Reiki Paths*, it's a straightforward procedure that utilizes the Reiki images for self-mending and keeps you concentrated on your objectives and dreams.

**Rundown**

There's something imperative to recall – Reiki is an all-encompassing practice. What's more, wealth, love or cash involves comprehensive methodology. That implies you can't generally draw in plenitude into your life if you center just around this little piece of your natural experience. You must improve your life as a rule – diet, connections, pastimes, physical body, profound convictions etc. Reiki encourages you to do this, obviously – Reiki heals each part of our lives. When we let Reiki do this, abundance will show itself. By mending our lives as a rule, we open the entryway through which plenitude really streams.

Did you realize that you can use Reiki and the Law of Attraction to help you get to your objectives?

## Law of Attraction and Using Reiki to Reach Your Goals

All you need to do to reach accomplishment with this method is to use it directly here, right where you are, right now. I suggest taking a shot every seven days, but you can pick what works best for you.

### How much simpler could that be?

Like I stated, this procedure that I'm going to indicate here uses the Law of Attraction combined with Reiki.

If you're inexperienced with it…

### What Is the Law of Attraction?

The Law of Attraction states that things, conditions and connections that fill your life are essentially the end product of the reflections, sentiments and energy you put out into the Universe.

Envision that there's a Great Big Cosmic Restaurant and you place your order (by how you feel and consider yourself and your life).

This restaurant takes in your order (the vitality that you've put out) and conveys back to you precisely what you've requested (conditions that match the sort of considerations, emotions and vitality that you have put out).

This Great Big Cosmic Restaurant doesn't pass judgment on you. It's not so worried about whether you're positive or negative, or in doling out remunerations or disciplines. It essentially gets your request as energy and sends back to you the related results.

The great news here are that by changing the energy you put out, you can change the nature of the things, circumstances and connections in your life. When it goes to the LOA - like pulls in like, so assuming you need positive things in your life, you must put out positive thoughts, words and feelings.

Bodes well, isn't that so?

**The Two Step Process to the Law of Attraction and Using Reiki**

**First:**

You're going to utilize the rule and standards of the Law of Attraction to help you set clear, well-organized goals in request to get what you ask for from your week ahead (or any time span that works for you) while starting to invest energy into showing them.

**Second:**

You're going to add extra, super-fueled indication power to the process with the assistance of Reiki.

Additionally, by utilizing Reiki with this procedure, you are going to be clearing ceaselessly any deterrents to your prosperity.

Both Reiki advantages are going to greatly increment the speed and success of your outcomes.

**Instructions to Use Reiki to Achieve Your Goals**

Like we've talked about, sending Reiki to your objectives is an incredible way to improve the results of most of your activities and work. Besides, if it's to your greatest advantage, it will even help to speed up your growth.

It will also help you end up mindful and break up any limits to your prosperity that you might hold within you. This way, the way to your objectives will turn out to be clear and simple, infant! What's more, as you've likely experienced before throughout everyday life, the less impediments you experience when accomplishing something, the simpler it is to remain motivated and continue onward. Talking about being successful!

Adding Reiki to the way towards accomplishing your objectives is likely one of the most effortless and ideal ways to ensure that you have the Divine assistance and support needed to transform your fantasies into reality.

We consistently have God or Spirit in our minds. Yet, except if we've requested help and intentionally separated the impediments to this help, we may not be getting the real accessible support that is waiting for us to take advantage of.

In any case, when we do this, most of the common help that we would ever need, in order to accomplish our fantasies reaches to us in the form of fortunate conditions and help from other individuals.

So right away, here are the means by which to utilize this:

## Stage 1: Write it Down!

First, write down your objective on a note.

You can likewise utilize a Post-it note or a note-taking application on your telephone. As we stated, you're going to need to ensure that you've expressed what you're hoping to accomplish both in positive terms and in the current state.

For instance: "I have the remunerating job I have always wanted."

At this point you can see how improving outcomes the recording: "I wish my activity didn't make me so miserable."

In case you're working with different objectives over the time of seven days, a month or more, you have two or three alternatives of how to approach the notes of your objectives.

You can either write them across the board rundown and put a heading at the top, for example "My Goals for the Week of January 1 through January 7," or "My Goals for the Month of January." And then send Reiki the gathering of objectives in general.

In case you're managing bigger objectives, you might need to record each one independently and send Reiki to them exclusively. In any case, you don't need to and it's alright to even now send Reiki to them as a gathering.

When managing day by day objectives, for facilitation, it's ideal to simply stay with one rundown of objectives and send Reiki to the group.

Another reward to this progression is that simply the demonstration of recording your objectives holds its very own specific intensity in helping you to accomplish what you want. What's more, interestingly, the vast majority never at any point get this far. You're now a long way on top of things!

After you record your objective, give yourself consent to feel a flawless little shiver go through you as you make magnificent things for yourself. Oooh! That is the inclination of progress!

**Stage 2: Add the Reiki Symbols for a Little Extra Oomph!**

Hold the file card in one hand, ideally your non-dominant hand.

Utilizing your other hand, draw the Power image over the card in light. You can also draw the Distance image and additionally the Mental/Emotional image over the card, as well, assuming you feel drawn to do it. Assuming you have other images that you know and use, you can include them, as well. In any case, just include the ones that you really feel attracted to. We're not going for a mess here. We're hoping to help and get clearness to the circumstances.

Assuming you are not familiar with the Reiki images or some other images besides, simply skip this step. It will thoroughly work even in this case. I guarantee!

The intensity of this method, while it is upheld and upgraded by the vitality of the Reiki images, isn't gotten from the Reiki symbols. It is your expectation, in addition to the Universal life power vitality that is Reiki and you, as the channel of this power, make the final product.

At this progression, you can also ask for the assistance and backing of any lead celestial hosts or rose masters with whom you work in accomplishing your objectives.

### Stage 3: REIKI!

Hold the record card between both of your hands now and give it Reiki for a couple of minutes (maximum 10).

The most effortless and best breakthrough ever!

If you're not familiar with Reiki yet, look at my answer for you towards the end.

Adding Reiki to the way towards accomplishing your objectives is additionally one of the most straightforward and ideal ways to ensure that you have the Divine assistance and support that you might need to transform your fantasies into reality.

### Stage 4: ACT

This progression is essential and not to be disregarded.

You need to take the steps required to accomplish your objective.

It's forced to think that you will accomplish your goals while sitting on the lounge chair throughout the day. This is a physical world and what we're living and the capacity to act is supported on this place. So, do whatever you can to help accomplish your objectives.

Since you've added Reiki to the blend, you will find that your achievements come much more effectively and with significantly less obstruction, both on your part just as from any other individual and that things simply appear to stream better. Impediments will essentially fall away, or their underlying forces will be uncovered to you so that you can discharge or mend them.

Likewise, ensure you're looking for indications of chances to follow your objective. Some individuals allude to these events as good fortune. However, whatever it is that you call them they are Reiki endowments and ought to be seized and hunted as the brilliant open doors that they are.

If it's not too much recollect that this progression is intended to enable, not to overwhelm. The activity steps that you might take will be Divinely guided now, accepting that you are tuning in to any direction you are getting.

You shouldn't work yourself to depletion to get things going. You might be called to buckle down, however more significantly, this is tied in with working more insightful.

Since one of the super-forces of Reiki is the creation and backing of parity, once you've added Reiki to your process, it will guarantee you balance.

### Stage 5: Repeat Daily

Same as you did in step three, give Reiki to your list of objectives for two to ten minutes consistently.

In the first part of the day, soon after you wake up, is an extraordinary time, as is evening time right before bedtime. Whenever it works for you and doesn't add to your pressure, but makes you feel bolstered and enabled, it's perfect for you.

If you need to, you can even bring the card with you so you can give it Reiki a couple of times through your day. This will help your outcomes and keeping you concentrated on your objective.

If you'd rather to do this, you may type your objectives in a note on your phone. Many of us have our telephones with us daily, you can give Reiki to your objectives at whenever you're holding your telephone. To do this, either open the note on the telephone or channel the energy towards the note while simply holding your phone.

## DO NOT BE DESPERATE, EXPECT CHANGES

Bringing this to a lovely point, below are some probable things you could come across while practicing this technique:

### Check it

You will probably see that you start to acknowledge better thoughts regarding how to accomplish your objective.

Your limits to your objective will likewise be mended.

You'll feel more and more motivated to accomplish your objective and become relentless.

You may even find that Reiki causes good fortune in your life and you will have the option to accomplish something far superior to what you've initially planned..

# CHAPTER 8
# THREE PILLARS
# OF MODERN REIKI

The Three Pillars of Reiki are: Gassho (Gash-Show), Reiji-Ho (Ray-Gee-Hoe) and Chiryo (Chi-Rye-Oh).

## Gassho

Gassho signifies "two hands meeting up". Gassho holds the aim of appreciation, regard, center, parity and association to collective awareness.

The Gassho hand position helps centering and calming the brain during contemplation. Place your hands in praying position with your eyes closed and carry attention to the tip of the middle fingers.

In a seated posture, place your hands in Gassho position.

Concentrate on where your two middle fingers meet.

Give your contemplations a chance to diminish.

## Discuss the 5 Reiki principles out loud or in your brain

Once you're done, express the intention of appreciation.

If you consider this reflection useful, it is advised that you perform it in the first part of the day and night for 15-30 minutes, in a perfect ambience for one month. You may think that it's important to keep track of your encounters, in order to reflect just as how your life circumstances change with time.

## Reiji-Ho

Reiji signifies "sign of the Reiki control". Ho signifies "techniques". Reiji-Ho consists of three short rituals that can be performed before each Reiki session.

Lift your hands in Gassho position, before your heart. With eyes shut, request the Reiki energy to course through you.

Request the mending and prosperity of the beneficiary. Lift your hands to your third eye and request to be guided to where the Reiki vitality is required.

Allow your hands to be guided. Disconnect from any doubs you may have regarding the result of the session and trust the Reiki vitality and your instinct.

## Chiryo

Chiryo signifies "treatment". Chiryo is performed by the professional holding their predominant hand over the customer's crown chakra and holding up until there is a sign to move, which the hand pursues. The Reiki expert keeps on utilizing their instinct considering the hand position until they feel the calling, as part of the practice.

The body and cognizance are associated by breath. We take in oxygen for physical survival and universal life power to feed and purge our soul.

**Two of the shorter reflection rehearses:**

Joshin Kokyu-ho is a useful breathing strategy for diminishing your pressure and refining your brain and body. It is likewise an incredible contemplation for both purging and healing.

Start in a to standing or sitting situation with hands in Gassho position. Close the eyes and inhale gradually, through your nose. Relinquish any pressure.

Hold your hands up as high as you can and envision the light (Reiki) showering into your entire body.

As you exhale, imagine that the light rounding your body is spreading out in every way, present and past.

Playing out this contemplation normally will reinforce your connection with Reiki. Some individuals, additionally discover that it increments their intuitive capacities too.

## Dan Tian

The Dan Tian is situated in the belly between the navel and pubic bone. The Dan Tian holds a supply of vitality. By setting aside some effort to interface with this vitality point, you can expand your imperativeness and guarantee you are a reasonable channel for Reiki vitality.

**Carry your psyche to Dan Tian and tune in to your relaxing.**

While you are breathing in, imagine that white light (Reiki) is filling your head and travels down the focal point of your body into the Dan Tian. Between each breathe in and breathe out, the light spreads to all pieces of your body. Feel that the healing procedure is continuing.

As you breathe out, picture that the light rounding your body is spreading out everywhere.

However, Reiki is an antiquated type of Japanese healing that is polished by numerous experts around the globe. There is a supreme energy that offers life to each living thing and the Japanese call this "Ki." It is otherwise called Chi by the Chinese, Prana by various Asian societies and most of the western countries refer to it as the Holy Spirit.

Chakras, a Sanskrit language word signifying "wheels of life," are vitality focal points found all through the body. The situation of every one of the major chakras relates with an endocrine gland or organ controlling hormonal balance. These Chakras are situated at the base of the spine (root chakra), between the pubic area and the navel (sacral chakra), two or three inches above the navel (sun based plexus chakra), the focal point of the chest (heart chakra), center of the neck (throat chakra), in between the eyebrows (third-eye chakra) and top of the head (crown chakra).

Chakras speak to explicit parts of the cognizant being and their primary capacities and attributes are the following:

## Root chakra

Color: Red

Body Parts: Adrenal organs, kidneys, lower area of the spine, leg bones.

Capacity: Grounds you physically.

Awkwardness: Afraid of life, confused, narrow-mindedness, inclined to savagery; low back, feet and leg pain.

## Sacral chakra

Color: Orange

Body parts: Gonads, prostate, reproductive system, spleen, bladder.

Capacity: Deals with imagination, sexuality and feelings.

Irregularity: Overuse of substances, sex or liquors; sexual or regenerative issues; perplexity, desire and confidence issues.

## Sun based plexus chakra

Color: Yellow

Body parts: Pancreas, liver, intestines, stomach, spleen, autonomic sensory system.

Capacity: Intellect and it is known as the source of individual power.

Awkwardness: Insecurity about monetary issues; need to control others; stomach related issue.

## Heart chakra

Color: Green

Body parts: Thymus, heart, lower lungs, circulatory system, skin, hands.

Capacity: Bridge between the physical and spiritual Universes; center of spirituality, prosperity and love.

Awkwardness: Sad sentiments, dread, outrage and possible coronary illnesses.

## Throat chakra

Color: Blue

Body parts: Thyroid gland, throat and jaw areas, lungs, vocal strings.

Capacity: Communication and mental inventiveness.

Unevenness: Communication breakdowns, excessive eating and drinking to keep away from reality; respiratory ailments, dental issues and low confidence just as outrage, antagonistic vibes and hatred.

## Third-eye chakra

Color: Indigo

Body parts: Pineal gland, lower brain, left eye, ears, nose, focal sensory system.

Capacity: Intuition and special insight;

Awkwardness: Fear of dreams, cerebral pains, sleeping disorders, tension and discouragement.

## Crown chakra

Color: Violet
Body parts: Upper brain, right eye.
Capacity: Direct association with soul.
Awkwardness: Loneliness, need to compare ourselves with others, fear of death.

By putting the hands over the seven Chakra points that are encountering any of the lopsided characteristics reminded and performing Reiki, these Chakras can be rebalanced, prompting wellbeing.

## REIKI AND CRISTALS

Accompanying Reiki vitality with Crystals makes them a powerhouse in mending your physical, spiritual and psychical body by accelerating the healing procedure.

Utilizing mending stones when performing Reiki makes an astounding joint of energy! They are incredibly compelling and, when put together, they work in concordance to enhance healing possibilities. It is accepted that the association between the stones and Chakras will restore the Chakra into a sound vibration, along these lines mending the part of the body more effectively.

## Reiki

Reiki Therapy has been around for many years and is known as Universal Life Energy. It has been perceived as coursing through every living thing and it's accepted to adjust our vitality stream and healing from inside.

Created by Mikao Usui, Reiki is utilized for the adjusting and blending of energies. It is most usually utilized in a type of treatment, from one individual then to the next to reestablish spiritual, physical and profound prosperity. Reiki can likewise be utilized to adjust the energies of creatures, plants, items, water and sustenance and so forth.

## Benefits deriving from Reiki

• Promotes Harmony and Balance;

• Accelerates the body's self-mending capacity;

• Dissolves vitality limits and advances characteristic harmony between psyche, body and soul;

• Assists the body in purifying itself from poisons and supports the safety system;

• Aids better rest;

• Helps to diminish stress and anxiety;

• Enhances positive energy;

• Lifts mind-set and clears the psyche.

## Precious stones

Precious stones convey certain energies and when they connect with our individual vitality fields or chakras, they can have a positive effect to boosting our prosperity and fitting our energies. Certain crystals help interface the vitality to our Chakras, which are vortices of life vitality. They work to associate the physical and spiritual components of our body.

## Advantages of Crystals

- Help in bringing abundance and clarity;
- Boosting vitality levels;
- Help us in not 'giving up';
- Promoting energy;
- Help to associate personality, body and soul;
- Help to counteract sickness.

Picking a precious stone that speaks to you...

Here are only some healing precious stones and their implications, find their properties and what they could help you with.

## AMETHYST

Gives unwinding, quieting properties. Allow amethyst's vitality of satisfaction to sooth away any burden that keeps you up during night. This precious stone works with the third eye and crown chakras. Amethyst encourages your body to have sound rest and unwinding and works with your third eye to offset the brain with wise answers for issues.

## AMAZONITE

Assuming your psyche is contaminated with dangerous cynicism, tidy it up with Amazonite. Severe mental distress we may have encountered in our past creates vitality obstructions in our present and this can translate in communication difficulties, problems when it comes to seeing someone or even in your work life. By filling your throat and heart chakras with cherishing vitality, this precious stone helps to open you up, to discharge what has harmed you so you can get rid of your issues.

## PYRITE

Generally known as "Trick's Gold" for its likeness to genuine gold, Pyrite is a magical fortune. As it helps in drawing in wealth and abundance, it is additionally accepted to hold a solid defensive energy. The intelligent idea of pyrite is something other than physical with its capacity to demonstrate to you which practices might keep you down, which make you increasingly mindful of what you have to change so as to vibrate the aim of abundane on a similar recurrence as pyrite.

## ROSE QUARTZ

Potentially one of the most prominent mending precious stones! 'See the world through rose tinted glasses' by taking advantage of the love of rose quartz. This stone opens your heart chakra to each sort of adoration that you need: love, fellowship love, familial love, love for humankind or sentimental love. As a flush of bliss, sympathy, pardoning, harmony and clearness beats through you, rose quartz will help you in discharging poisonous feelings so your soul can at long last be free of cynicism.

## TIGER'S EYE

This crystal's capacity to initiate fierce concentration and basic power reflects its tiger-like appearance. Tiger's eye moves your standpoint so you can increase a more profound comprehension of yourself. Is there a piece of you that you need to analyse? Another leisure activity you might want to try? An answer for an issue you haven't considered? Something you need to do or see? Tiger's eye interfaces with the sun based plexus and sacral chakras to give you the power to seek these callings.

## SUNSTONE

Similarly, as the sun carries life to all the living things on Earth, Sunstone will revive your innovative soul. It advances vitality, inventiveness and imperativeness. Its radiating vitality helps you to remember the delight in making and motivating. Sunstone supports the sacral and sun based plexus chakras to breed certainty, power and initiative. Free from underneath the cover of self-question, your innovativeness will at long last thrive with the intensity of the Sun.

## SMOKY QUARTZ

This gem doesn't have the sort of vitality that is going to give you a chance to sit in a dim, dull room and sulk. Smoky quartz will assist you with getting up, attract the blind to positive light and open the windows to give the demeanor of antagonism a chance to get out. Working with this lovely gem helps you defeat negative feelings, for example stress, desire, dread, outrage and even sentiments of wretchedness. Elevating your mind-set with this stone encourages you to stay adjusted and positive in any circumstance.

## RHODOCHROSITE

The self-esteem precious stone that will battle sentiments of deficiency, lifting your spirit and giving you a mindset of self-esteem. You deserve the adoration you get and Rhodochrosite energy causes you to acknowledge that by topping you off with affection and delight for yourself. This gem of strengthening works by injecting your heart chakra with the fortitude and inspiration to take on new challenges. Give unequivocal love a chance to overwhelm any sentiments of bitterness.